SOUND MEDICINE

HEALING WITH MUSIC, VOICE, AND SONG

by
LAEH MAGGIE GARFIELD

CELESTIALARTS
Berkeley, California

CELESTIAL ARTS
P.O. Box 7123, Berkeley, California 94707

Cover Art from *Celtic Stencil Designs*, copyright © 1990 by Co Spinhoven
    New York: Dover Publications, Inc.
Cover Design by Toni Tajima
Drawings by Gabrielle Gern and Pam Yates
Singing for our Lives, Words and Music by Holly Near © Hereford Music
    All Rights Reserved
We Are the Flow, Words and Music by Shekhinah Mountainwater
Back Cover Photo by Lorri Goodman

Library of Congress Cataloging-in-Publication Data

Garfield, Laeh Maggie.
    Sound medicine

    Includes index.
    1. Sound–Therapeutic use.   2. Music therapy.
I. Title.
RZ999.G315   1987   615.8'5154   87-13223
ISBN 0-89087-483-2

First Printing, 1987

Manufactured in the United States of America

3   4   5   —   96   95

Dedication

For my grandchildren.
Whether they're born into our family or brought in
through love, this book is dedicated to you with
great hope for the future of our world.

— Oma Laeh

ACKNOWLEDGEMENTS

I wish to thank my parents Lawrence and Doris Garfield for their invaluable help proofreading. A soupçon of thanks goes to Lianne Wolf for fulfilling the role of archivist. Nancy Schluntz, my trusty editor, who finetuned the manuscript, deserves much gratitude. André Christiaan Cuppen, thank you, for translations of Dutch and German, and for tooling around Europe with me as I researched and wrote. Heartfelt appreciation to Bob Wachtel for supplying the computer wizardry that made a friendly user out of this former computer wimp. Recognition also goes to Samuel Spitzberg and Rabbi Hanan Sills for their hours of help with Judaic research. Without Iris Ostling and Sandra Pastorius, the readers who aided and abetted this project, this book would be the poorer. Praise also falls to Anna Kealoha, musical transcriptions; Gabrielle Gern, line drawings; Trixie Robinson, levity; and Mary Ann Anderson, typesetting and layout coordination, and all the tiny details that make a manuscript into a book. I am indebted to Jack Grant, who supplied sage counsel and encouragement as only a professional writer can. Plaudits also fall to Kari Clark for extraordinary patience in bearing with me through two completed books and several in progress.

Multitudes of thanks to David Hinds who fostered and supported my efforts to set flight as a writer on my own.

Seventh
(crown): universal consciousness, mediumship [pituitary gland]

Sixth
(third eye): intuition, creative insight, clairvoyance [pineal gland]

Fifth
(throat): communication, clairaudience [thyroid gland, brain, eyes, ears, nose, mouth, bronchial tubes, esophagus]

Fourth
(heart): personal love and universal compassion [thymus, heart, lungs, shoulders]

Third '
(solar): power, energy, [adrenals, liver, gall bladder, stomach, blood and lymph]

Second
(sacral or splenic): emotions, security, clairsentience, [pancreas, kidneys, skin, uterus]

First
(root): grounding, survival [ovaries or testes (fertility), large intestine, bones]

LOCATION AND FUNCTION OF THE SEVEN MAIN CHAKRAS

TABLE OF CONTENTS

INTRODUCTION

I see my work as demystifying the mysteries, making the occult or unknown available to the masses without obtuse language. In the clearest, most practical manner possible, this book seeks to reveal the deeper levels of the psyche which we are all privy to, yet the majority have been taught to deny. Taking the lid off the pot to see what's cooking when it smells good is everyone's desire. Unfortunately, there are many sanctions against exploring the myriad realms of consciousness. Despite this, millions of people are examining their inner experiences and setting out on quests for more. They read multitudes of books written on anything esoteric, study the ancient religions, searching for enlightenment, and meet with like-minded others. These people are the change makers who wish to go forward with life as spiritual warriors, taking the inward journey as their challenge in life.

There isn't any point in maintaining esoteric secrecy. It hasn't made our world safer to have mystical knowledge in the hands of a self-selected few. Occasionally some demonic leader has taken charge of sacred sites or occult knowledge and abused them, but ultimately their meanness is their seed of destruction. When more people know healing and occult methods for transformation, the greedy ones who rule our current world will have less opportunity to preempt the available resources and energy for their own private

1

plutomania. The purer our thoughts are, the less likely we are to wreak havoc in the world.

Basically, anyone has access to mystical and spiritual knowledge. The majority only require reassurance and some assistance to recognize their own experience as mainstream mysticism. Mystical occurrences have not varied that much throughout the ages; only the social language they are couched in has changed. Every faith, at its core, bares the same rich experiences for the ones who are willing to risk all and follow their hearts. The wondrous thing our time offers is that multitudes rather than a circumscribed few can find their own pathway to higher consciousness.

To become one with the mysteries of life and the universal laws, you must learn to listen in a new way. When you have an unusual visionary insight, trying to bend or mold it to fit into your current operating values and belief systems is futile. You have to set aside many of your cherished beliefs and grow others. Sometimes this means you will feel empty for a spell until the knowledge has integrated itself into your life. Seasoning is an important part of Truth and right action.

Essie Parrish, my mentor, who was a Pomo Indian shaman, spent a lot of time talking to me about attitudes and people's life stories before she stirred in esoteric information that I could recognize as such at the time. She forbade me to take notes, teaching by repetition and memorization. A subject would come up numerous times; each telling contained a few more salient facts. One day she gave me a significant look and said, "To get a special Healing Song I had to go up to Mt. Shasta on at _____ site, and sit four days in _____," which meant, Now go up there and do what I told you to do. Indian people are indirect by Anglo standards of communication. I had learned to listen in a non-European way, to know when she gave me detailed information about making preparations for myself, an exact location, or that this vision quest could only be done at a specific time of year. If this was that season, I should make arrangements to do it immediately.

I became aware of my Lifesong about a year before I met Essie Parrish. It'd played me, by singing itself inside my head, while I couldn't call it up if I wanted to. The Universe chose the times it was available to me. Due to its intensity and power I was continually enchanted by it. At first I didn't know it was a Lifesong since it had come to me spontaneously while I was journeying on the inner planes. By the time I met Essie Parrish I knew what it was and how it functioned. When she asked me to, I sang it to her in confidence and she nodded that this was indeed my Lifesong.

We all have equal access to these shamanic, creational mysteries, but most people cannot receive them without adequate information or preparation. The purpose of writing Sound Medicine is the same as when I wrote *Companions in Spirit*. Readers are looking for ways in. They seek simple, practical, down-to-earth methods to further their inner explorations.

Sound Development

The auditory method was not my main means of ascertaining spiritual knowledge. I was not clairaudient except in unusual circumstances. Therefore, the development of vocal healing was a complicated project for me to undertake, in contrast to colors and emotional "knowing" which came easily via clairsentience. I could walk past a building and smell, taste, and feel what was going on inside. If I wanted to know something, telepathic images (clairvoyance) would appear. To this day when a person comes for a reading I simply turn on the movie and watch the screen in my third eye.

You've probably known students with photographic memory, who are always out having a good time and getting straight A's as well. That was me in every other area of the medicine path. Discovering how to work with sound was a major achievement. Essie Parrish, my teacher, couldn't push me far enough, fast enough. There was a brick wall around me concerning sound. When it came to making sounds out loud with and for clients, I was tremendously inhibited, just as most of you are. There is also a barrier within our culture about making sounds. Overcoming it is one of the greatest challenges of working in the medium.

In 1976, I finally capitulated and devoted myself to exploring the potentials of healing with sound. It was complicated for me to learn, which is why it is one of the easiest things for me to teach. I had to open to it step by step by praying over it, asking for it, falling into it, meditating, and taking prolonged inner steps.

That summer, while my children busied themselves with friends and country activities, I sat for hours contemplating properties of sound beneath the naked ear's hearing. In silence I sought sounds I'd been told about but never heard. From the stillness arose the primordial sound, the song behind God's breath, which holds the

Universe together. It rose in my throat and poured forth, to my own disbelief. It was another year and a half until I was satisfied this sound was correct. Out of doors in the cold December air I sang it loud and full, knowing it was perfect. The high-pitched, resonant, dramatic soprano sound came octaves above my usual vocal singing range.

After a few months of exploring variations on that form of sound, I discovered which sounds worked on each chakra. Tentatively, I began to sing these sounds for clients at the end of a healing session. The results were beyond my wildest expectations of how powerful a renewal is possible through sound. Experimenting further, I taught these musical intonations to my class. They were elated by the power of their own voices and the cacophony of sound that become one sound, one consciousness, as they each sang separately in the room. Later I learned this form of sound is called *Svaha* or Esoteric Sound or Toning. This type of high tonal chanting is used by medicine people in sweat lodges, ceremonies, and other ritual healings. So important is the high-pitched quality of the chanting that Native American men chew a horribly bitter root to help their vocal chords achieve it.

Some of the sounds the book will introduce to you are tonal qualities I channeled myself. These won't be familiar sounds from other sources because it was apparent to me that in a society based on passion, greed, and envy, a different set of sounds would be required to alter and raise the vibration of each chakra. Openness to tuning into to a more refined system of sound healing yielded an unusual combination of vocables.

One May afternoon in England, a woman handed me a yoga book by a renowned but publicity-shy swami who resides in the Los Angeles area. He too uses the sounds I've found via the "Universal radio station," and for the same reasons. There truly is nothing new in the entire Cosmos, only the continual rediscovery of what the Universe, or the Source, has already delivered to our plane of existence. Our skill in catching the information correctly allows it to work properly or to be incompletely understood.

Somehow I have tuned into the things other mystical seekers have learned. When it turns out that different people have been given the same information, it serves as confirmation. You may learn many things from many authorities, but do your own explorations as well. Continue to educate yourself, practice frequently and examine what is correct for you. Eliminate what is not working, irrespective of where you learned it. Sometimes this means you're not ready for the practices and can incorporate them later. But it can also be that the source of your teaching was faulty.

A well-appreciated musician went on a vision quest with a person who teaches shamanism but is in no way a shaman. The musician received a song on her quest which she wrote and recorded on an album. Her teacher had failed to tell his students not to reveal their Lifesong. Perhaps he was unaware of the precaution. Three months after the album was issued, the singer contracted a fatal disease. She had given away her power by recording that song and letting others sing it. The most horrible thing to me is that the group leader is still out there in his ignorance, dispensing and playing with sacred knowledge he knows all too little about himself.

The directions for exercises have been painstakingly perfected, some over centuries, and some by me through trial and error singly and with students. You should follow them to the letter to avoid difficulties. On a warm spring day in the early 1970s, I was practicing the Meditation of Water detailed in Chapter 11. Nearly an hour into the exercise I fell over backwards, breathless and drained of all energy. Not only had I failed to take a break at the appropriate time, but I wasn't aware of the need to cover my head once removed from the water's edge. Stubbornly, I pushed myself upright and began to meditate, and rapidly collapsed again. Fortunately, a wise spirit guide instructed me to lie back and rest before proceeding. Later I learned to cover my head between segments of this meditation.

If this text says never to do something, *then do not ever do it*. Precaution is better than repair or regret in the case of exercises or meditations. In healing, the one who makes the sound can be wounded from it as well as the person it is intended for. If done in innocence, then the Universe will be kind and make the correction for you. A deliberate misuse of a technique, however, is noticed by the guardians of sound and will at some time be paid for. The same is true of forbidden sounds or ones which must be used with caution. I've already broken some taboos to see if they truly were dangerous, and ascertained that the spirit allies and my teacher were telling the truth. There's no need for you to throw a lighted match into a gas tank to see if it will ignite. Should you be the curious type who absolutely must see for yourself if this is true, attempt it on your own headache, indigestion or any simple, minor ailment, which can later be remedied with aspirin, Maalox, peppermint tea and other non-toxic home methods.

The human body has an extremely low frequency rate of eight hertz. This is close to the vibratory rate of our Earth 7.83 hertz. Competent healers automatically attune themselves to this vibration. They do this by breathing in unison with the client, thereby restoring the out of balance person to the correct hertz level. This recreates body, mind, and spirit harmony.[1]

Commitment

There are levels of initiation which cannot be given until you are ready and have done the necessary preparatory work. There are also things which can only be transmitted teacher to apprentice in person. If you aren't ready to receive and assimilate the information all effort is wasted on you. When my teacher, Mrs. Parrish saw that I was willing to commit my life to this work she gave me the sounds to call the helping spirits.

Throughout the text, exercises, ideas, and methods are expounded at length, not to titillate you, but to assist you in your growth. Assimilating esoteric material is beyond thinking: your heart and soul must interact as well. If you read Sound Medicine strictly from an intellectual viewpoint or perform a practice once or twice and forsake it, you will have little success. Diligence is the true mark of anyone wanting to become competent in any field. Mastery of sound, earth, water, air, fire, or healing is not to be dabbled with and abandoned. These are serious studies which must be learned from the inside out. No one can give you their expertise. Esoteric matters are always personal and the experiences you have defy linguistic descriptions. We both may be awestruck listening to someone sing their Healing Song, but the impact varies according to what each of us brings to the moment. Your entire personality and belief system affect your perceptions. Therefore, as you practice these methods your rate of evolution depends upon your rate of commitment. As in the example of a ham and eggs breakfast, the chicken is involved, but the pig is committed. Commitment is the single most influential ingredient in spiritual growth. Without it, you're just another tourist exploring the inner landscape.

---

[1] See Chapter 5 for an explanation of hertz.

1
SOUNDING OFF

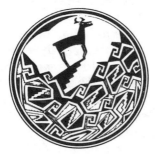

Sound Body

Absolute silence is foreign to all of life. Even when we are vocally still, our bodies are always making sounds. There are digestive sounds: belly rumbles, passing wind, swallowing, food gurgling as it goes down, gulping, burps, lip smacking, and teeth clacking together. We make breath sounds: snorting, sneezing, wheezing, inhaling/exhaling, sniffing, blowing the air passages clear of mucus and irritants, panting, and snoring. Internal and external movement sounds accompany us moment by moment: our heartbeat and pulse, joints cracking, the pounding of our feet on the ground as we walk, our hands tapping and slapping against objects in our daily tasks, finger snapping, fingernails scraping, jaws clicking, teeth grinding, clothing rustling, and hair singing when it's clean and wet. Human beings are not quiet creatures.

Our mouths and vocal chords emit releasing sounds: moans, groans, grunting, snickering, tongue clacking, mmm, shushing, heavy breathing, hissing, giggling, laughing, pleasure moans, heaving sighs, yelps, shrieks, yawning, raspberries, sobbing, crying, sexual sounds of ecstasy. All these expressions without words indicate pain, pleasure, joy, sorrow, exertion, and the full expanse of human emotions. Our voices range from a whisper to ear-shattering cries.

These sounds are natural expressions universal to people in every culture regardless of language. Yet we have been taught that all of these sounds are either impolite or ought to be suppressed except under very special circumstances. The sounds of lovemaking communicate your needs as effectively as carefully chosen words. Allowing involuntary vocal expressions to flow lets your partner become more attuned to you. And your mate's sounds help you to be a responsive lover as well.

There is such resistance to letting out sound that healers and therapists must continually encourage their clients to make the ones they feel. People lay in hospital beds after surgery in tremendous pain and stifle their moans. While still a youngster, you are told to act maturely and cease exhibiting emotion publicly, especially crying. Yet crying is an essential ingredient for health maintenance. Scientists examining the tears of people crying from emotional pain have discovered chemicals in them that differ from those shed while peeling onions. People who cry have fewer stress-related diseases than those who limit expressing feelings that trigger tears.

Soundview

Sound is the energetic force field that holds our galaxy, the Milky Way, in orbit. Everything in the universe has a vibration, a tone underlying its beingness. Planets, stones, plants, animals, the wind, water, fire, earth, each contains an indigenous tonal expression characteristic of its energetic framework. Every human being has a distinct sound wave permitting us to recognize those who are known from outsiders. Even inside a family or tribal group an individual's sound or vibration distinguishes them from their look-alike cousins.

Sound classically produces a strong alteration of consciousness, notably heightening the senses and meditative states. The reaction to music and natural sounds like waves breaking against the shore, coyotes or timber wolves howling, strikes a chord in our psyche that reaffirms our oneness with the Creator and our own world. When repeatedly confronted with displeasing sounds, we tend to withdraw from life as well as the discord.

Sound judiciously used is far superior in alleviating psychological pain than all the legal and illegal drugs Western society has toyed with. The high produced by sensitive listening becomes an enduring quality one can turn to whenever the mind or body requires renewal.

Synesthesia

Synesthesia—the blending of senses—is most frequently and powerfully triggered by sound. A precise sound or musical piece may bring visual images into our mind's eye, set off olfactory sensations, or evoke taste. Sound can touch off a series of memories or take you into the future. Visual imagery can produce taste, smell, and sounds no longer heard in the world, such as the voice of a deceased person. All of the earthly senses can singly or in groupings bring out the experience of the other senses so vividly that we are in the moment they occurred rather than in memory.

This process defies verbal explanation. There is no reason hearing a steam whistle makes you smell pancakes or picture a 1961 Buick. Touch, as in lovemaking, may also produce visual stimuli. During or following orgasm people sometimes have glimpses of past lives they shared with their lover. Sound, when it delivers you to memories, creates sensations in the body that induce involuntary movements. These twitches, chills, shakes, finger and foot tappings release joys, sorrows, and fears that haven't been fully discharged.

Synesthesia, a natural, inborn, intuitive phenomenon, is almost always pleasurable. It's somewhat akin to telepathy, with which we all begin life. Yet only ten percent of the adult population has sensory crossover. Children, with few exceptions, experience synesthesia regularly, but it vanishes in the socialization process. We do children a disservice teaching them not to tune into a multiplicity of senses at once. Adults challenge them with statements such as, "You're only seeing a photograph. There's no music here." Those hardy souls who have kept their aptitude intact into adulthood are to be congratulated for their fortitude and self-possession.

To regain your full sensory capacity, isolate yourself either with headphones or by taking private time to listen intently to some of your favorite musical pieces. It may take several weeks of experimenting with the lighting, whether the room is lit or dark, and the type of music you're playing. It's easiest to start with something you were very fond of when you were young, like the Beatles or the tune that you shared with your first romantic love. Close your eyes, breathe deeply, let yourself relax totally so your mind floats freely as you hear the music. Let your consciousness float, meandering until you reach smells, sights, and memories which are more real than ordinary recall. Continual reconnection with synesthesia in a specific setting will set the stage for spontaneous experiences.

The Fifth Chakra and Health

Sound is one of the three major creational and healing forms. It came before Light and Breath (prana), if you believe the first paragraph of The Gospel According to Saint John: "In the beginning there was the Word (sound). And the Word was with God, and the Word was God." Sound is related to the fifth chakra at the hollow of the throat. Clairaudience (inner listening) is its intuitive form. Light is related to the sixth chakra, often called the third eye since it sits invisibly between the two ordinary orbs in the human face. Clairvoyance, (inner sight) is the gift Light bestows. The heart chakra is the seat of the breath or life force (prana).

The wheel of energy called the fifth chakra is vital to our mental and physical well-being. Through it, we express our truest reactions to life. Particles of non-material matter enter and leave our throat chakra as breath and sound. When we lie or deny what we feel with spoken words, we are destroying our own body/mind. It is extremely difficult to be honest at all times. Although we may wish to speak the truth, employment, the health or feelings of another, or our physical safety deter us. Deception and deceit undermine the functioning of the rotating energy wheel known as the fifth chakra. A sore throat is a negative experience brought to the physical body as a way of telling us we are out of balance. Physical ailments also serve to clear negativity brought in by dishonesty, listening to lies, speaking falsely and maliciously, battering another by speaking harshly without sufficient cause, or being verbally abused ourselves. Even when called upon to reprimand another person, it is best to speak only of their detrimental acts and not assassinate their character or attempt to destroy their self-esteem. Truthfully and tactfully said, whether to a child or an adult, constructive criticism is most productive and least destructive to yourself and the other individual. After all, as the cynical spiritualists say, "What goes around comes around." If we deliver a severe verbal dressing down to someone, in time the venom rebounds, often from an entirely unexpected source.

Your Word is Your Fire

Words have power to heal, help, create, irritate, detract, or destroy. Careful use of speech is one of the most important parts of spiritual development. As you learn to manifest energy and increase your power, words that harm come back at you in one form or another. Mrs. Parrish always told me not to gossip. There is a vast distinction between malicious talk and trading information. Telling a neighbor that someone has a beautiful garden with extra vegetables to share is fine, unless they've asked you not to let others know. Keeping secrets is an essential part of judicious speech. On the other hand you're not doing a teenage alcoholic a favor by keeping their public drunkenness from their parents. A good rule to follow is to ask yourself what your intention is in speaking about someone. If it is to cast a shadow on their reputation or make yourself look good by comparison, silence is the best discipline for your own growth.

Individual words can be very powerful. Years ago Mavis, a wise woman, was brought to my house. She worked for the Red Cross disaster team. Her life was full and she appeared to always have what she wanted. She taught me some key words for fulfilling needs. They've worked very well, although I don't know the original source. Mavis had learned them from someone else. They are:

Find. Money
Reach. To locate lost or misplaced objects or to reach a solution.
On. To get transportation when you need it.
Clear. To get clarity in a situation.
Together. Main switchword for all things that need to happen or be restored to balance.
I am. Oneness with the divine.

Words carry energy in their intonation, strength of delivery, and our emotions at the time they are said. In ordinary use the same word, phrase, or sentence can be interpreted as an understatement, overflowing with praise, or sarcastic. What we say not only has ramifications for the listener but for ourselves as well. It is vital to begin each day with cheer and good words to set the best prospective tone for the day. If we use grumpy or deriding words first thing in the morning the entire day may be a spoiled mirror of its beginnings.

A student of mine called upon her best friend to complain about a neighbor first thing in the morning. She'd had a tumultuous series of interchanges with the neighbor over the past few months. Vilifying her, spreading her anger out, my student felt better when she parted from her friend. A while later she bumped into an old friend. He began a tirade against a false guru and several business competitors. My student, disgruntled by all his detrimental talk, attempted to change the conversation to another topic, to no avail. Her friend persisted in mocking others. She extracted herself from their chance meeting as quickly as she could, but she'd lost three-quarters of an hour. Her head felt fuzzy and she was a bit disturbed, so she went to a favorite coffee shop to relax. There she encountered a colleague of whom she was quite fond. He sat with her, his conversation discharging all his frustration and anger about their department chairman, who was going through a personal upheaval that seeped into his working hours. My student, remembering that your own words set the framework of the day, knew she had somehow called for this lesson to illustrate the point. But, she asked me in desperation over the phone, "How can I stop it?" The answer I gave her was simple, "Laugh. Tell the next person you see funny stories that ridicule no one. Laughter breaks the cycle of negativity, and shared laughter all the more so."

Naming

My mentor, Essie Parrish, always said never to name a disease since that will give it power over you. Clients bring me a diagnosis and I tell them to forget it and what the words mean, since knowing how an ailment progresses isn't necessary to develop all the symptoms and complications of it. Everyone has complete inner communication and can, even unconsciously, tune in on all the thoughts that have accumulated about an illness. Manufacturing a sickness is only a matter of thinking of its name in connection with yourself and in due time you'll have it well underway.

A famous dance therapist came to me for a reading. He was healthy, but overworked. My advice included hiring an administrative assistant to free up his time. This he did, but he also assumed new projects. Fifteen months later while on tour he was hospitalized. The diagnosis was AIDS. He died within three months from the dreaded malady, although tests run on his cadaver showed no trace of the disease or its related sydromes. After I returned to the United States many friends and students of his came to speak with me. They were terribly disturbed that he'd died of an unknown illness (very likely extreme exhaustion) that was misdiagnosed as the still "incurable" AIDS.

Names

The very names we are called by our friends and family affect our thinking about ourselves and how we are perceived by others. Every name carries its own energy and beliefs that go with it. In his study of eight hundred common names, Christopher T. Anderson, author of The Name Game (Simon and Schuster 1977), surveyed college students to ascertain what they believed about specific names. Spelling and sound, nicknames and full given names each were assigned different meanings by the respondents. Males and females reacted somewhat the same to the majority of the names. This sampling will give you an idea of the impression a name conveys: Ann was judged ladylike, honest, but not pretty, while Anne (the same name with an E) was beautiful, sociable but untrustworthy; Dave equaled a superstar, a he-man and an achiever, and David was not quite as terrific as Dave but still an undeniable winner; Mark and Marc were both considered spoiled; Katherine was determined, strongwilled, and comely, and its diminutives were similar—Kate, unstoppable, and Kathie, very likable; John was trustworthy, surprisingly passive, but very manly, while Johnnie was a winner across the board; and Jack, diligent and very sexy.

Numerous studies have sought to determine the effect our names have on us, some concentrate on our overall characteristics and some to predict popularity and success in later life. Children who have pleasing names that aren't overly adult sounding are much more popular in day care or other early childhood school settings than children with difficult to pronounce or tonally harsh names. Therefore Willy might be better liked than William and Casey more accepted by his peers than Cassius. Nicknames must change as we get older so they fit who we have become. Adults over six feet tall called Shorty, a real estate agent named Trixie, or a Mrs. five-by-five nicknamed Birdie are at a disadvantage.

Multitudes of people aren't fond of their names and this affects their personalities as well as their relationships with others. There is nothing wrong with renaming yourself; many people do just that. Johnnie becomes Jack, Concheta becomes Connie, Bobby decides to be Rob, Maria opts for Moira in modifications of the original name. Many people are more fond of their middle name and become R. Sonya Smith, rather than wear the loathed first name evermore. You can also completely change your first name if you so desire, using your birth name only on legal papers. You can adopt any given name or surname or both just by consistently using it without intent to defraud. Or you can change it legally. This is a simple procedure requiring a lawyer and some time; however, it is permanent, and all your documents will reflect the change.

In many tribal cultures children are given a "milk name," which is changed in puberty or later once the individual has endured a challenge or otherwise shown what their true nature and capabilities are. A technique no longer in favor was used in Eastern Europe by Jews whose relatives were ill. They would change the person's name in order to confuse the bad forces that were looking for them. Surprisingly, the method often worked, with the full knowledge and consent of the sick person, because it changed their own inner harmony and outward vibration.

Part and parcel of the identity crisis many women experience upon marriage is the impact of changing her name. While the majority of women wish to be Mrs., they are not aware of the vibrational change a new name bestows. Your energy has been ruled by the name you bore as a maiden. That name is swiftly removed at the wedding and a new one substituted. The welcomed name is not familiar when linked with your own first name and many brides do not respond when a caller addresses them as "Mrs. Brown". They still resonate with their previous name. One good way to limit the extent of the crisis is to keep your own name or to retain it at work. Then there will still be places where the sound of your name keeps your old self at a functional level.

Singing

Singing for medicinal and spiritual expansion takes a multitude of forms. The lost art of singing has been relegated to church choirs, operatic performances and the entertainment industry, but everyone can sing, tap their feet or fingers, hum along or drum. The human form lends itself to making music. The voice box was and is the first wind instrument.

Singing is one magnificent way to discharge unpalatable emotions. It is better to chant or sing away the blues than to permit desperate feelings to disturb your life. Singing cures the spirit in a way that drugs cannot. Songs in songbooks are very reasonable to buy, or you can memorize ones you like from the radio. Writing the words to melodies you like in a small notebook can assist your memory when learning a song. Tape recordings and records help as well. If you are shy or easily embarrassed and worry about your voice quality, play the recording by your favorite singer and sing along with it until you're brave enough to go it alone. Don't fret over losing a note or two or going off key. When the mental or emotional state you're in clears, you'll sound as good as or better than Johnny Cash. Singers practice their numbers for hours before performing. Why expect first-night quality when you're just opening up to the dynamic energies of your own voice?

Chants for removing depression, expressing joyousness, averting danger, better concentration in meditation, and other benefits are practiced throughout the world irrespective of culture or sophistication. They help balance your emotional, physical, and mental state as well as opening up the spiritual pathways. Many people who enjoy chanting or singing regularly gather with like-minded others. Glee clubs, local plays, senior citizens centers, and parties all provide opportunities for songsters to sing.

Songs are linked to memory. Any information put into rhythm or music makes an indelible impression on our minds. This accounts for the success of commercial jingles. Many of our earliest rules of written language are taught to music. Who doesn't remember the order of the ABC's or the months of the year by the ditties sung about them?

Throughout this book you will be instructed in minute detail in vocal formats for healing, gaining insight, and spiritual growth. You don't have to be gifted musically to learn and perform these songs. The only requirements are an open heart and an open mind, coupled with perseverance.

2
VOICE AND SOUND

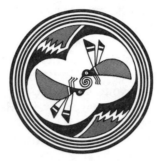

The Voice

"After death only the voice will be the same."
Essie Parrish, Pomo shaman

The voice is a measurement of the developmental level a human being has achieved. The voice is our breath, the essence of our very life, our being, with sound added to it. The voice is therefore our truest mirror of inner health, mental stability, or lack thereof, emotional excitement or disinterest, and spiritual attunement. The tonal quality of our speech tells more about us, on a subtle level, than the words we say. And often, if the voice isn't balanced in the right manner for the subject we are speaking about, our words will be ignored.

A great part of our personality comes through the voice. Sound gives away our true intentions as well as how we feel about ourselves. The healthy person has a well-modulated, clear, rich, voice that is kind in tone and word. The wispy voice of a shy person, the cracking voice of someone in fear or under tremendous stress, and the booming tones of someone who is trying to put one over on you are all dead giveaways. The rounded, sonorous sounds of a person who believes sincerely in their projects and follows their inner light is quite different from the indwelling abrasiveness of the super salesman who only wants you in their grasp 'til the money is delivered. The voice of someone who isn't quite sure what they are speaking about projects only uppertones and is devoid of undertones. Accomplished actors have learned to perfect these subtle qualities in delivering their dialogue so that they are convincing as the characters they play.

The voice gives evidence not only of what you are sending out, but what you can take in. A closed person has a stern, resistant voice. The voice demonstates how deeply you explore life and how well you assimilate fresh concepts. A thin, tired voice shows someone who doesn't have energy and interest in life. An underlying whine discloses a generalized unhappiness and dissatisfaction with life originating in early childhood. Flat tones equal a life sans excitement; a hysterical delivery denotes fears. Clipped, short speech indicates a curt, impatient personality. Mellow, honeyed tones reveal the savoring of joy and vital interest a multitude of experiences have brought to bear on the individual. A raspy voice can mean the person is tired, and sleep may help alleviate their unpleasing-sounding speech. Oftentimes the person with severe stress has a grinding undertone to their ordinary speaking voice. A sweet, sunny voice that is natural rather than put-on reveals an optimistic person. The voice of an older smoker, with its pleasantly suffocated median range, points to illnesses soon to emerge from the complications of tobacco use.

The individual who has lost their voice due to laryngitis is unable to recover from extreme fatigue. Speaking builds body heat, and when a person is listening only for another opening in conversation to talk again, the heart rate accelerates rapidly. The body's response is aphonia, removing sound from the voice to quell the overabundant heat built up by excessive talking or competitive social interaction.

In addition to the mental and emotional attitudes already outlined, a lack of depth and breadth in the voice betrays physical infirmities. The absolute indicator of the voice is its timbre, which makes it instantly recognizable as the voice of a single person and no other. Timbre is the characteristic quality of sound produced by a particular instrument or voice. If that changes, the person has suffered a significant contrary impact to their health and well-being.

The Tibetan teaching of *zDzogChen*, or the Great Perfection, considers the human being to be made up of three interlinked patterns of activity: the body, the voice (vital energy), and the mind. When one is ill or injured, Tibetan physicians say the problem is due to disturbances and imbalances of the person's body, voice and mind.

Afterlife contacts with deceased persons bear no resemblance to the infirmed voices of illness nor the one they had immediately preceding death, unless they died of accidental causes while apparently in optimum health. Instead the discarnates have their own voice at its best, representing the highest growth and integration of character achieved in the lifetime. If their voice consistently had mellifluous tones, then that is exactly what you will find. People whose hoarse, muted, sharp, or edgy voices were their norm, still speak in that manner years after their passing. The person speaking from the other side will use a vocal pattern and timbre that was their own at whatever stage of life you knew them. Should you have known them over an extensive time, they'll pick the voice most familiar to you to communicate with.

Learning Communication

Speech is a special skill learned through our earliest contact with other fully socialized beings. A child who isn't spoken to and is isolated from speech during the first few years of life will be unable to develop much of a vocabulary, or may not be able to speak. The way we relate verbally to newborns, three-month-olds, six-month-olds, year-old babies and two-year-old youngsters varies automatically. As the child grows, the mother (usually) and others close to the child use varied forms of soothing speech, which prepare the little one to talk. The mother and/or father speak to their infant with vocal tones and specific sounds indicative of their language to gently coax and assist the baby to hear and then mimic structures and habits of sound. Primarily this prepares and allows the child to form sounds, words, and later sentences with creative and individually varied usage of their mother tongue. This process exists in all countries, in both civilized and native cultures. It is known as Motherese*. We learn it from our primary care person and pass it on to our children instinctively. All the intervention of competent speech pathologists cannot make up for the lack of consistent talking a parent does while holding and cuddling their young. The development of hearing is also linked to the skill of Motherese a babe is exposed to.

---

*Jan Vorster, Lingua, December 1975

Second Languages

Children are completely capable of learning two separate languages and distinguishing between them. Bilingual families have successfully imparted fluency in both languages simultaneously to their youngsters.

A family of my acquaintance with an American father, a Haitian mother and a Mexican housekeeper taught their toddlers three languages at once. The children became adept at speaking English to the father, French to the mother and Spanish to the housekeeper. If they spoke Spanish to either parent, neither would answer, although each knew the language well. The children were free to converse in any language amongst themselves and sometimes used all three when at play. They were quick to size up which language to use with a new guest. Since our worldview is governed and colored by our language, these children (now adults) have a wider horizon than single language speakers.

Languages, through what they include and exclude, prearrange the depth we can get to in a particular area. In English the word statue signifies a three-dimensional piece of artwork, but isn't indicative of what it is. *Standbeeld* literally means standing picture in Dutch, leaving no doubts.

Since the mid-1960s, words have crept into English concerning states of consciousness our native tongue couldn't articulate. English and its nearest linguistic relatives, German, Dutch, and the romance languages, have borrowed the same words freely from Sanskrit and Tibetan. *Karma*, meaning intention or conditions responsible for ones fate, *prana*, meaning life force, and a multitude of other words and phrases have been integrated into our languages so we could discuss spiritual matters more fully. Prior to the adoption of these foreign terms, the English speaking mind, without words to communicate, couldn't fathom the variations meditation and inner visions made in our consciousness.

Standard wisdom claims it's not possible to adequately learn a foreign tongue when you are over forty or grown up, depending upon whose narrow view you accept of your own intelligence. You may make mistakes characteristic of non-native speakers with American, Canadian, or English background at first. And you may talk with an accent either slight or marked, but you can become fluent. Given enough practice in the language, surrounded by native speakers, you may even lose your accent. The more you practice, the more you visit sections of cities or the nation(s) where it is spoken, the more adept you will become. As you attend movies or theater in that language, you'll assimilate its tonal qualities and nonverbal communicative forms.

Pick your teacher carefully. Choosing someone with whom you have rapport is an important factor in learning another tongue. This teacher is your new parent, who is doing a version of Motherese with you. Enroll in a small class that specializes in speech, rather than reading or writing the language.

The best way to learn another language as an adult is the "look and hear" method. Seeing the word in print is extremely helpful to the literate person. Have a native speaker pronounce it for you. Say it again and again until you get it right. There are tones you cannot distinguish without repetition or unless you retrain your ears. Observe closely the mouth of the person talking to you. The shape their lips form and the placement of their tongue, the throat or nasal sounds they make as they speak will all become part of your subconscious knowledge about your new language. Listen carefully in a relaxed manner and don't hesitate to ask the other person to talk more slowly because you are a beginner. Play that role for as long as you really need it. Don't pretend to comprehend what you cannot understand. Straining to hear is self-defeating and distorts the facial muscles, cutting off aural sensitivity. Therefore, listen and breathe slowly and evenly, following the conversation for as long as you can. Breathe deeply and continue listening for words and phrases you're already acquainted with. If the topic of conversation is known to you, you're more likely to follow it even if you don't actually know all the words.

Imagine yourself as a foreigner learning to hear the difference between close sounding English words such as vary and very. To learn a second or third language means taking risks, being a child again, adapting and surrendering to the experience of listening with both your inner and outer ears. Realizing it takes a baby at least two years to master its mother tongue to the point where anyone can understand him or her, will give you an idea of how long it'll take you to become an expert. Much of the progress in a new language is by osmosis. Flow with its richness and the sounds will become ever more familiar to you. Success will come earlier if you are learning a language you heard your parents or grandparents speak or if you're highly motivated by a career or personal interest.

Once you are able to speak, do so with minimum stress. If you can talk for only half an hour without becoming tired, stop then. Your endurance will improve as your sentence structure, idiomatic expressions, and love for the language increases. On days when you are stressed or ill, the new language may appear to vanish and you'll remember little of it. The less tense you are, the better your health is, the easier you will be at thinking, speaking, and listening in your new language. One night you'll wake yourself up by dreaming in that tongue, and then you'll know you are proficient.

Deafness

There is a vast difference between being born deaf as opposed to becoming deaf. Deafness at birth is usually a karmic learning experience sought by the soul. When it proves to be surgically remedied, as in the case of overgrown adenoids, the requirement was temporary. However, many forms of deafness are currently uncorrectable and the individual must learn about communication in other ways than speech. That is the challenge of their lifetime, and fortunately many master it so well it no longer presents itself as a handicap. Parents and others close to the child are also required to make accommodations which will enrich their lives and provide them with lessons of the psyche and spirit. The deaf have great telepathic capacity, sense of smell, touch, taste and keenly feel sound via vibrations. Frequently they comprehend the world via the three senses of intuition: clairvoyance, clairsentience, and clairaudience. Their experience of the latter is via thought forms beyond words. Deaf children born to deaf parents have instant communication, whereas deaf children of normal hearing parents have a tremendous barrier to overcome.

Obstructed hearing can be due to environmental factors, physical disease, or emotional distress. Partial deafness permits limited communication and asks for more intense listening from normal hearing persons. Speech may be slurred or contain nasal tones. With proper counseling or some of the latest technological advances, the hard of hearing can communicate effectively.

Children who live in a home where there is incessant bickering often decide to close off their ears. The deafness is psychological and not physical, but the results are just as devastating. The cure is to have the parents learn communication techniques so that the fighting is ended. If they cannot do this they're best off separating in the interest of every family member's mental and emotional health.

In later adult life, seventeen percent of the population suffers some degree of hearing loss. Many of the hearing-impaired people I see have spouses who talk incessantly, or they've been one-half of a pair of fighting partners. Others barely speak and live alone in near isolation aside from their jobs. Some people who are going deaf never listened to other people anyway. They made up their mind in advance and kept themselves walled off from hearing another's opinion. In this type of deafness, the mode of living is mirrored in physical limitation.

A colleague sent me her eight-year-old son who was deaf in one ear and had a slight impairment in the other ear. The child had a speech problem as well. I already knew that the boy and his step-father were at odds. Whenever the boy attempted to tell a story he would get through the first few sentences normally. As he progressed he would go faster and faster until his words became a muddle of saliva and poor pronunciation. He was anxious about losing his audience, but his dysfunctional way of dealing with it lost them any-way. He went into his pattern as he told me a story. I listened intently, yet he did not perceive that he had my full attention. I stopped him and told him to begin the story again and to clasp his index finger with his other hand. This time he told the entire story with deter-mination and a normal, even delivery. At the end he looked at me and said, "Is that all it takes? Do you mean if I hold my finger I can tell a story?" Worry can be stopped in any situation by grasping the index finger. It works to ground a person. In the boy's case he needed it for self-confidence.

His next problem was more difficult to remedy. There was no way to keep his stepfather from being verbally abusive. Although many states have laws preventing physical cruelty to children, none have programs to deal with psychological battering. As is usual in childhood deafness, extreme fear was affecting his kidneys. He also suffered from anxiety, which taxed his spleen. His mother was will-ing to use herbs to cure him with the understanding that it would take several months. Juniper berries were recommended and the boy bravely drank the strong decoction. The berries were simmered in boiled water for twenty minutes. He used about three cups (70 mil-liliters) per day. Other herbs that remove fear from the kidneys are stinging nettle and red clover in combination. These are simply taken as a tea.

A woman in her late sixties came to me with a vexing hearing loss. Occasionally she lost her ability to hear for a few hours. Lately it'd become annoying as she'd lose a conversation midway through only to have her hearing return to normal after several minutes' interruption. A long-distance swimmer in her youth and still swimming daily, she used ear plugs to keep water out of her ear canal. I suggested a mild solution of vinegar to wash the inside of her ear, suspecting she'd acquired a fungus. One teaspoon in an ounce (30 milliliters) of water is sufficient. I told her to keep it in a brown dropper bottle and apply it with the dropper several times a day. She was skeptical and went to her doctor, who advised the same remedy be tried before more stringent pharmacological measures.

In determining whether a person is nerve deaf or if the cause is repairable, stand behind them with your open hands three inches (seven centimeters) from their ears. Bring your hands in close to their ears and pull them out again several times. People whose hearing loss is temporary, repairable, or psychological, will have strong waves of energy usher forth from their ears in response to the stimulus provided by your hands.

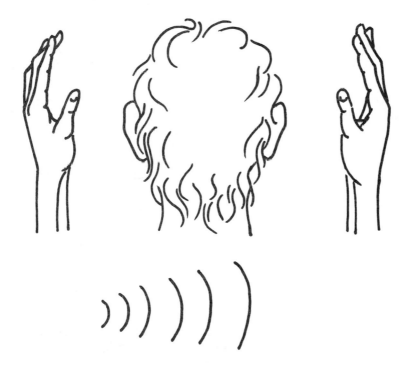

To stimulate the return of normal hearing function, hold your hands as described on the previous page. Begin with a small circle and spiral clockwise outward using a conical formation. Do this five or six times in succession. Stop for five minutes and repeat. If the volume or tone of hearing is greater after this treatment, the person can regain most of their original capacity with proper diet (no sugar, no dairy* products) and regular use of Toning and Overtones as instructed in Chapter 5.

Health care professionals ought to do this treatment every time they see a client who has the potential to recover from hearing damage. The client can receive more regular help if a cooperative friend or member of the client's family is taught how to do it.

Voice & Song

Voice is a universal method of releasing in song. If you can speak you can sing. Carrying a tune isn't a prerequisite for expressing the happiness or monotony of your life through music. Many a homemaker hums a little tune as she works, relieving the sameness of her work. Those who work alone or have to drive long distances can utilize this system of alleviating boredom, enjoying a reverie, blowing off steam, or sweetening an already beautiful day. My Aunt Rose would hum tuneless tunes while she hung out her wash, and the troubles of people who'd come to see her earlier in the day, for the sage advice and counsel she offered, vanished.

It is well established that families who sing together harmonize better in other ways as well. Mothers driving their children to and from after school lessons or errands can sing with them. The children are humored and amused, and singing effortlessly stops them from harassing one another. School buses filled with singing children have fewer difficulties, as the songs uplift the spirits of the non-singers as well. Nonsense songs children learn from one another are perennial favorites.

Cowboys sing to their cows to keep them together. Swiss farmers have a special whistling melody to call cows at milking time. On long journeys to and from the summer mountain grazing area, they yodel

---

*Milk products impede healing because they're poorly digested by older children and adults. Dairy consumption is always contraindicated for healing.

to keep the cows moving along placidly. The herd reacts quite favorably to human vocal chords vibrating musically.

The origin of yodeling, it is said, was to make the mountain spirits friendly. Who hasn't whistled as they walked down a dark alley to allay their own fears or perhaps to keep trickster entities at bay. Exorcists sing and chant to clear homes and remove possession. The Alphorn, a beautiful, deep, resonant instrument whose sound vibrates throughout your body and psyche, was played morning and evening in former times to sing to the saints. Therefore we can assume that vocal musical expression has powers to charm beyond the physical realm we live in.

Keening

The human voice can powerfully change our circumstances, creating harmony or sending an opponent reeling. Shouting from the guts, a custom of karate, is a perfect example of the latter. Keening, also called wailing, is a type of singing that discharges sorrow.

Keen is from the Irish Gaelic, caoinim: to wail or bewail with a keen like a widow bereft; to make a sound like screech owls. A lamentation or dirge for the dead uttered in a loud wailing voice; a lamentation or cry of grief; a rhythmic recounting of the life and character of a dead person.

The word wailing comes from the Scandinavian weilen: more at woe; to express mournful sorrow audibly, make mournful outcry, lament, weep; to make a sound resembling or suggestive of a mournful cry.

A keener is one who keens, especially a professional (usually female) mourner at a wake or funeral.

Keening was restored to the modern world by the women at Greenham Common, England, who wailed for the state of our planet, as its people enveloped it in the making and deployment of arsenals of death. Prior to reinstituting this method of grieving as a political protest, only aboriginal peoples and professional mourners of particular ethnic groups in industrialized nations kept the ancient tradition alive. Mothers in Ethiopia and the Sudan were seen on television during the famine of 1984 emitting wailing sounds over the bodies of their children.

The sounds themselves are piercing, and rip away the hearer's facade of emotional control. Wailing women who surrounded the

Pentagon at the lunch hour in a 1982 demonstration so disturbed the war-minded gentlemen who work there that they shrank back into the building rather than penetrate the wall of sound.

In practice, keening is a melodic, mournful combination of a moan and a cry done in unison or with overlapping waves of sound. Worldwide it comes from the women's culture. In George Gershwin's Porgy and Bess, Bess lets out a stylized form of Wailing in the song, "My Man Gone Now": oohoohoohohooo.

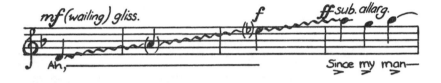

Keen Instructions

First do these exercises to relax your throat and diaphragm. Go through the chakras, reciting E for the first, O for the second, I for the third, U for the fourth and AH for the fifth. Breathe inward and let the sounds come from the different chakras. Feel the vibration. Then put the sounds together in this order and sing it like a siren: E-O-U-AH-I-E-O-U-AH-I- continuously.

Gabrielle Gern, of Lichtensteig, Switzerland, who wailed with the women of Greenham Common, made the following commentary. "Start with AH, then do a few siren sounds to find your pitch. Then stay in that sound range and wail; don't force it. Send the energy to where you want it to go. I was surprised at how easy it was to direct energy like this. And I was amazed how I suddenly knew when the keening in me had finished. I didn't feel empty, but the energy to send out had been spent. It was rounded off. I kept breathing deeply and felt how clear my body was inside. Clean and straight."

She also offered this partner exercise to help loosen you up before keening with a group: "Your partner stands behind you, arms encircling your waist. Bend over slowly, vertebrae by vertebrae. Touch your hands to the floor if you can. Your partner bends their knees so you can almost sit on them. Relax, allowing your partner to rock you gently from side to side. Make any sound you feel like and let it come from deep down inside. That will relax your diaphragm. Come back up slowly, breathe, and change positions with your partner."

With many voices keening together, they each begin at a different pitch and remain that way for some time. When the group is better than midway through they begin to blend their wailing, falling into the same octave and rhythmic pattern. The majority will also trail off together, some ending in low moaning sounds and others in a great series of exhalations. Then the group is very still and little activity occurs for a few minutes. After that there is often an eruption of smiles and laughter.

Keening can be done singly or in groups. It's a grief sound without sobs or screaming. While the sound itself brings up sorrow, it prevents hysteria. Gently bending the knees and swaying back and forth assists in clearing out old griefs or a current shock. Keening can become rather loud and disturbing to the neighbors, so it's best to do it indoors during hours they are gone. Showers are a great place to let it all out, as is any flowing body of water. The sounds of the water also serve to cleanse your heart and soul of past pain. (See Chapter 11 for a fuller explanation of the healing powers of water.) Keening is especially good to do in the car while driving, for that is an isolated, very private space when there are no passengers.

Once you permit yourself to keen adequately and long enough to release old unhappiness and sorrow, you are ready to partake of the joy and pleasure your current life offers. Painful times buried long ago will disappear without effort or psychological counseling when you adopt keening as a healing method. If you are in the throes of a recent death or loss, wailing will help you through the process. You will still experience denial, anger, depression, and rationalization, but in the end acceptance will come much sooner.

Keening is always performed early in my Sound Medicine classes to enable the attenders to enjoy the rest of the material offered. It frees everyone emotionally and aids them in becoming a cohesive group. Participants feel as if they've unlocked doors of intimacy with the others, when not a personal word has passed between them. Sorrow is discarded without the instance of deprivation ever hitting the conscious mind. This technique makes singers out of the inhibited and helps in locating the Healing Songs and Lifesongs.

When keening you use a large amount of liquid. Put your hand in front of your mouth and exhale several times. Unless the weather or your house is especially dry you will feel quite a bit of moisture on your palm. Emitting sounds utilizes moisture laden breath. Half an hour of exhalations such as you've just done would require rather a lot of fluid. It is wise to drink plenty of water or herbal tea before and after keening. People who suffer from water retention will find the quantity in their tissues diminished by wailing. The effect is much more lasting than taking diuretics. Retained body fluid is cast off in the release of emotional tensions.

Singing Over Plants

Traditional cultures varied in approach to harvesting wild plants. Native peoples in each area had different procedures to honor the plant's spirit, i.e., leaving an offering (corn, tobacco, sage or cedar leaves) while others sang over plants. The songs for gathering herbs are highly specialized and divergent from tribe to tribe. There are songs for blackberries, songs for sacred root plants, songs for slippery elm, rabbit brush and other medicinal plants. As the women collected, peeled and prepared the roots, seeds or leaves of herbs and trees, they sang. Each herb in some tribal cultures has its very own song which you must know and sing to take part or all of it without offending the plant's guardians. Rather than attempt to teach the "right" song for each plant, connect with the Cosmos and you'll be given the one you are to sing over it.

If you wish to find a song for an herb, sit quietly in a secluded location without touching it and respectfully ask that it teach you its harvest song. For some, the answer is rapidly delivered; for others, the wait is long. When the spirits of the plants know you are sincere, the information is forthcoming. Sincerity includes not drinking, smoking only when the spirits tell you to, abstaining from recreational drugs, being clear of purpose, and spiritually caring. A student asked if recreational drugs included sacred herbs or mushrooms. If you take them reverently on occasion in a spiritual manner for the sole purpose of gaining inner knowledge, then they are consumed respectfully and with honor. You don't need sacred herbs to be given the songs. Meditating or merging with the spirit of the plant usually produces results. Harvest songs can also come through drumming.

Although the drying procedures and care shown in storing may be equal, plants that are sung over at the time they are gathered last longer than ones which are plucked from their growing places with quiet reserve, and the latter retain their potency longer than those that are taken in haste with no thanks offered at all.

In the early summer of 1977 some friends and I were visiting eastern Washington. When the man we were staying with found we were interested in herbs, he announced that he had a lot of mullien growing on his land. Mullien is good for coughs and bronchial problems, can be smoked instead of tobacco in ceremonies, and has a multitude of other uses.

Although the leaf size and the length of the stem may vary due to factors like sun, water, and soil, the healing properties remain the same. These plants had exceptionally long, thick, leaves. They virtually covered the entire ground between the house and the creek.

Standing amongst them I offered a prayer to the guardian spirit of the plant and began to sing a sweet soprano melody that floated octaves above my normal vocal range as I gathered. We weren't able to be as careful with the plants as I like in our crowded car, driving fourteen hours to reach home the next day, yet the plants dried to perfection, never minding their rough treatment.

Three years went by. I was teaching at an herbal college and it seemed fitting to offer the students some non-technical advice on the gathering of plants. Sweeping three jars out from under a cupboard (which is where herbs ought to be kept, safe from the harm light does to their viability), I packed them into my assortment of samples for the class. During the morning session the three jars were passed around for the students to identify: which one had been picked this year, which the previous year, and the one that was old. They incorrectly selected the three year old mullien that had been sung over as the newly harvested one. The others jars of mullien had been gathered without their song.

A student who lives in Portland asked, "How can I dry and preserve plants well after I've sung over them?" "Your car is an Oregon dryer," I answered. For those who live in damp climates, spread a clean blanket or sheet across the back of your car or station wagon. Lay the flowers or herbs on it so they aren't touching one another. Close the car and park it in the sunshine; if there is none, leave it in an open place during daylight. Eight hours later you will have dried plants.

Singing Over Food

One truly important observance Essie Parrish taught me is to sing over food to purify it. You can sing your Healing Song, a favorite hymn, or a chant. You needn't sing it out loud if it's not convenient.

During the preparation of food, the person cooking mayn't have been feeling well. The cook might have been angry or upset, and that energy will go into the food. In big groups or in restaurants people tend to seize their food without a moment of silence or any thanks. Since you don't know what went on in the kitchen, or what the field workers and shippers were thinking as they handled the food, stop a moment to sing over your food or purify it in silence by giving thanks.

At a potluck supper there are three similar chicken salads. You're attracted to one over the others. Perhaps that one was made with love and truly offered to the group while another was grudgingly given. Every sound remains in the food whether our physical ears can hear it or not.

Attitude towards the food is equally important. If you choke it down saying, "This is good for me," when you don't like it, or you spend two days apologizing to your body for stopping at a fast food place, it'll have an adverse effect. It's not so much what you put in your mouth, it's what comes out that creates a favorable climate for health.

3
MUSIC

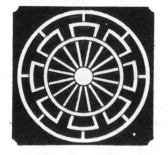

Most of us listen with half an ear to music that isn't our favorite type, while songs or arias you are drawn to captivate your entire mind. You listen raptly to them. When the car radio is playing a thoroughly revolting song, the flick of a switch replaces the sound. In a public place where you cannot turn the dial, you sometimes feel ill or trapped by the music.

Music is powerful as a tool to control mass consciousness and behavior. National anthems unify the people of a nation. They are meant to inspire loyalty to the country. The intention of religious music is to bring the congregation to a hallowed, pious state, opening the followers in awe and wonder to what the pastoral staff offers. Sounds sacred to one religion are often incomprehensible to those unfamiliar with the music.

Some spiritual music has merged into popular culture outside of its own religion. Black gospel and spirituals lend their enthusiasm and soulfulness to blues, rock, Motown and rockabilly, to name a few. Hindu chants and ragas have worked their way into folk songs and rock music in addition to becoming a revered art form of their own in the West. Cultures intermingling with North American and European society have brought their musical heritage to bear. Indian music from the entire Western Hemisphere has had a deep and binding influence on our own. Jazz, an artistic form imitated throughout the world, is an outgrowth of African music, reinterpreted by black musicians. Isolated in hostile white America, they founded a musical lineage that has outlived legal segregation and will outlast racism.

We are not only exploring other cultures musical roots but our own. Rapid alterations in our society's language and writing style that took place in the mid-sixties markedly changed our music along with other art forms. Motifs foreign to Westerners have been incorporated into our popular music as well as symphonic works. There has also been a revival of Renaissance and medieval music in recent years.

Music is so universal that it affects human beings irrespective of their race, ethnicity, religion, or political affiliation. Music breaks down the barriers authorities build, just as those in power use music to retain the status quo. Innovative, clear-sighted people, outside of the mainstream, have played music that eradicated entrenched powers. From time immemorial, philosophers have believed in the hidden powers of music.

"The persuasive and mathematical purity of harmony in music inspires the hearts of the listeners in a mass experience. The forceful mystery of this tonal relationship can be demonstrated as an invisible language altering our perceptions of reality. The profound experiences of art, education, healing, religion and patriotism are expressed in music. People are inspired, in times of harmonizing, to feelings of universal perfection and truth. Confucius said: "Those who can wholly comprehend this sacrifice can rule the world as though it were spinning on their hands."

The Pentatonic Scale is common to all folk music. There are only five notes: the fourth (fa) and seventh (te) notes in our ordinary scale are skipped. Oftentimes, if you are in a mild trance state you cannot tell Irish folk songs from Greek ones . The music isn't the same rhythmically or in topic, nor are the words alike, yet there is something indefinably akin. The underlying humanness in all types of folk music shows we are all related to one another at the core, though our ethnic mannerisms and beliefs change from one geographical area to another. Before people became musically sophisticated, their channeled music and the things they sang about were similar. The infinite forms music has taken throughout the ages is indicative of the level of sophistication of the civilization that supports it, as well as the spiritual attunement of the musicians who play and compose it.

From the I Ching Workbook by R. L. Wing, Doubleday & Co. 1979.

Chakras and Music

Every chakra is affected on multiple levels by music. Depending upon the chakra you are nourishing in your life or the chakras you are avoiding caring for, you are attracted or repelled by music that touches that chakra. Frequently, music you were enchanted by at one period in your life, you later revaluate as empty or irritating. Other types of music continue to sustain you and supply comfort throughout your lifetime. Categories of music which have been ignored due to unpleasant sensations experienced on first exposure, can become the mainstay of your listening once you and, sometimes, the musical style have matured.

If you're a person who is too open in the sixth and seventh chakras you might feel overwhelmed by fifties style cool jazz and therefore avoid all jazz. New Age music, which soothes the sixth and seventh chakras, is heavily endowed with soft types of jazz, comforting to spiritual seekers. To avoid overstimulating the root, sacral, and solar chakras, shield yourself from snappy, loud, upbeat, music with juxtaposed rhythms and melodies, such as boogie woogie, hard rock, and heavy metal. Instead you can find solace in music characterized by slow, predictable, repetitious, harmonious sounds, like chamber music or music for easy listening.

Reggae music lightly taps on the second and third chakras, gently caressing them open. Hear it and you are lifted along, despite any resistance to growth and change. Drumbeats of more aboriginal derivation work their magic by opening the entire chakra system. The beat works on sacral and throat first, then moves to root, and heart; returns to two (sacral) and five (throat) again, zeros in on number three, the power chakra, then proceeds to the linkage of one, four, and six. Only after the seasoned drummers have unveiled these energy centers does the rhythm approach the much guarded crown chakra. Like a charm it works to take the listeners and the drummers themselves into deep trance states wherein contact is made with the Creator. Adept rock groups and especially gifted muscians can mimic these techniques to give their live audience a shot of the cosmic stream in concert. The most exceptional ones will transfer the same energy to their recordings.

Classical composers Bach, Beethoven, Vivaldi, Mozart, Handel, Dvorak, Copeland, Sibelius, and many of their contemporaries wrote music capable of transporting audiences to realms of consciousness far above their daily lives. Each symphony, tone poem, opera, choral or concerto works on several chakras during the length of its performance. The listeners are really moved, some to great emotion, by the music. Because classical music usually contains a story of mythic proportions or is an ode to God, it crests and falls; themes and subthemes repeat throughout. Many works have an overture, which introduces the musical panorama prior to the main body of the composition. The pieces contain either spectacular dramatic endings or soft ones that seductively lead you back to earthly reality. Classical music has withstood the test of time and is well attuned to its audience. It delivers fresh insights with every hearing. The composer themselves may have been ahead of their time and little appreciated for jarring the sleeping multitudes into higher planes of self-awareness and contact with the source.

In popular music, salsa is one of the most dramatic innovations. It functions in the same manner as classical music. Salsa, however, within a few notes jumps from the first to the seventh chakra, clearing each one in the process and leaving the listener in a freer and more creative mood. Naturally, people flock to hear it, as it erases bleak emotional states and brings a joyful mood.

Concertgoers will notice that each conductor places their own stamp on the works being performed. Some can elevate the orchestra to peaks of inspiration, taking the listeners along as well. Avid rock fans eagerly assemble to hear their favorite band play renditions of other musicians' works. If you listen seriously to how another singer delivers a song you'll notice that it may effect you in a completely different chakra. For example, Bob Dylan and Joan Baez have recorded many of the same songs. Most people agree that his version is felt in the first chakra while hers touches the heart chakra.

These examples are just to give you an idea of the broad subliminal influence of music; even background music lightly listened to, imprints a tremendous reaction on the body/mind.

Some forms of music work on specific systems in the body. As an example, soothing, soft music is best for eating and digesting. Music with sudden bursts of sound stimulates the nervous and hormonal systems. Blues banishes downward mental conditions. If you pay attention you will feel energy running through your kidneys or circulatory system while certain forms of music are playing. If you have a heart condition, by all means, permit soft uplifting music to heal you. Notice not only if you enjoy or dislike a piece but if it has benefits you can feel while listening.

Yehudi Menuhin in his book *The Music of Man* (Simon and Shuster, 1979) describes music: "The emotions which music arouses grow out of something the Germans call *bermut*, that profuse, extravagant abandon which we associate with spring, with love, and with passion. Music is a measure of the powers that inhabit us, be they beatific or demonic, and which we try to keep in balance and to which sometimes we yield."

Music can sway our senses, take us to the brink of insanity, or shatter our illusions and leave us in the cold dawn of self-awareness. Notes held within us that are wrong for our harmonic field can do great harm, whereas notes or chords that resonate correctly with us restore health, hearten us, and inspire the courage to live life fully. We have scant knowledge of the Greek musicians who were able to know a person through a single note. Legends survive of these great healers, who could tune into the inner harmony of an individual and then play one note on their lyre, which totally healed their patients. It is said that if someone knows your sound they can control you with it. Sadly, most of us don't know our own sound or possess the wisdom to avoid songs that are harmful to our sensitive contact with our higher self.

Basic Music Theory

Ali Akbar Khan, a leading master of Northern Indian music, is described by Alan Watts: "Comprehension of music is understanding one note. He can sit for hours working on only one note at a time. He gets into that note and listens. He really listens, gets into the sound. It simply doesn't matter that it takes a long time, that he has to do this for many hours because he's completely absorbed in listening to the sound he is now making. He's going on with that vibration, as when you chant as they do in yoga AUM. You can chant for hours and be absolutely fascinated by the vibration." *The Essential Alan Watts* (Celestial Arts, 1977).

Like Bob Dylan, I cannot read or write music. Unlike Dylan, I'm unable to compose. What I've learned has been from dancing, singing, and inner knowing.

Cindee Grace, N.D., Phd., devised some theories about healing with sound published in issue 39 of *Well Being Magazine*. The excerpt offered here is a concise readable explanation of music theory taken from her 1978 article, Music and Healing:

All music consists of pitch and rhythm. Pitch is how high or low the sound is; how fast or slow the air is vibrating. The faster the vibration, the higher the pitch sounds to us. We perceive pitch because our ears register the vibration in the air, water, or whatever substance is carrying the sound waves. If the vibration rate is slower, the pitch sounds lower.

The letter names A, B, C, D, E, F, and G, are used to label specific pitches in traditional Western music. Other areas of the world notate music differently, and some types of experimental Western music also communicate with symbols other than these letters. But most music, from classical to rock use the principles outlined in this section.

These letter names repeat themselves over and over again. Each pitch is higher than the ones before it.

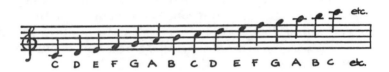

Rhythm indicates how long (in time) a pitch is sounded. Each pitch, randomly arranged in a song, can be of the same, or different duration than its neighbors. Actually, individual pitches are called "notes," and the duration of a note is called its value.

Notation	Name	Rhythmic Value
o	whole note	four beats
♩	half note	two beats
♩	quarter note	one beat
♪	eighth note	one half beat
♩.	dotted half	three beats

A flag put on a note cuts the value of that note in half: an eighth note is really a quarter note with a flag. It is half as long as a quarter note, because of the flag that is attached. Two eighth notes equal one quarter note. Sometimes notes have a dot after them a dot adds half the value to a note.

Usually, each song or piece of music has an overall rhythm. The word "rhythm" most often refers to a certain, repeating pattern of strong and weak beats.

In a scale, notes are arranged in successive order. It begins and ends on the same letter name e.g. (C-D-E-F-G-A-B-C). In addition, the pitches in the scale must be a certain distance apart, in terms of vibration. For example, the vibratory difference between C and its immediate neighbor D has been labeled a "whole step." Whole step means that the space between C and D is a measurable distance. The distance between any D and its immediate neighbor E is also one whole step, the same identifiable unit. However, not all distances between neighbors are whole steps.

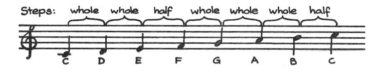

No matter the note duration, no matter where notes are positioned in a song, E and F are half steps apart, B and C are half steps apart, and the other notes are whole steps away from their own neighbors.

To satisfy the requirements of a scale, the notes occupying slots three and four must be a half step apart, and the two notes in slots seven and eight must also be separated by a half step. Luckily, if the scale begins on C, the slots are filled correctly.

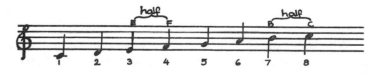

But suppose we started the scale on another note, G for instance? Remember E and F, along with B and C are always half steps apart.

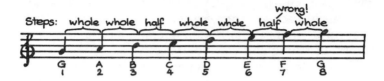

How can this scale be salvaged? Easy! By raising the F one half step (F sharp) we open the space between slots six and seven and make a whole step where one is needed. And that same action closes the gap between slots seven and eight, creating a half step.

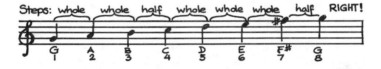

In any scale, notes can be raised (sharp) or lowered (flat) to insure that the proper relationship within the scale is maintained. Sometimes, the natural half steps (E and F; B and C) find their way into slots three and four, or seven and eight. When they don't, we can correct it by sharping or flatting the notes.

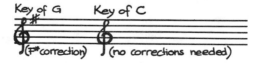

Whatever note fills slot one is the **key note**. In the last example, G was the key note: therefore, any music based on the G major scale is in the **key of G**. You could expect F sharps throughout the songs (unless changed by the composer's whim back to F natural) Instead of writing in a sharp sign at every F, the composer places the F sharp at the beginning, in the **key signature**. This sharp means all F's are sharp.

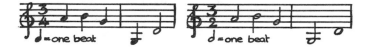

That's what keys are all about! They are based on a scale beginning on a certain note. These keys are similar to Pythagoras' modes and each scale has a unique effect on the physical, emotional and mental well-being of a person.

Time signatures tell which overall rhythm continues through a piece, just as key signatures indicate which scale. The top number is the number of beats per measure. The bottom number shows what type of duration gets one beat.

You may recall the chart displaying the types of duration (whole note half note quarter note). If the bottom number of the time signature is four, it means that the quarter note equals one beat. If the number is two, the half note equals one beat.

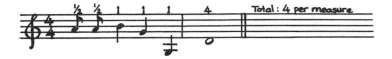

It does not matter how the indicated number of beats per measure (top number) is arrived at, just as long as the note values add up to that top number.

Anyone Can Play Music

In the previous chapter vocal musicianship was shown to be universally available. There are some instruments that even the musical wimp can play. These instruments are uncomplicated, sound charming, and do not require years of work to relish your own playing. Bells, tambourines, drums, spoons, and other simple instruments are open to your evolving talent. All you need do is practice, experiment, and risk the joy of learning that you too are musically inclined. Please restrain yourself from indulging in excuses about how you were born an inharmonic clod. You may be repressed, but you're certainly capable underneath your fears.

The drum is very likely the simplest of instruments to pick up and play with feeling. You mayn't evolve into a master, but you can easily learn to keep your own rhythm. Begin with ONE-two-three-four and repeat, emphasizing the first beat. If you fall off rhythm, just begin again without fanfare. When you have the four-beat down pat, you can double the timing, changing the accent to one-TWO-three-four or one-two-THREE-four and experiment in other ways. Additional ideas about drumming appear in Chapter 4.

Bells of various styles are either struck or waved in a circle. You can use the four beat idea of the drum, ring constantly, or play different size bells, which emit distinct notes. The main consideration is to let yourself become part of the music and permit it to move you along.

A tambourine only needs to be held in one hand and shaken to the beat of music played by others. You can shake it with the hand holding it and strike it with your free hand. All these instruments are open to experimentation. Whatever you do is the right manner to play them. The simpler the instrument, the better, until you develop confidence.

Adults needn't be timid about taking lessons on the trombone, flute, or piano or forego any other cherished idea of playing and playing well. Due to their intellectual advancement, adults and teenagers progress rapidly, provided they practice regularly and attend classes.

Channeling Music

All the music ever written has been channeled. The very nature of music is spiritual art, repeatable, uplifting and ever changing. The composers whose works have endured for several centuries were master psychics, or channels, who attuned themselves to the entities who set the stage for future human development. Many never were famous or successful in their own lifetime. Others were acclaimed, then relegated to mothballs until a later generation ready for the keys to universal wisdom rediscovered them.

Primary channels are composers who listen with their heart and inside themselves find a fragment of inspirational music upon which they build a song or an entire symphony. There are times when a song arrives full-blown, without a note requiring any changes by the alert, active channel. This opening into Cosmic Consciousness is the same one very advanced healers and prophets receive information from.

A Secondary channel is a musician who, hearing something that another person has composed, finds a thread in it that lends itself to the construction of an entirely new piece or is blended into the new composition. The composer many times will credit the work as based on a refrain of Claude Debussy or another musician he admires. Of course there are the copyright violators who chip pieces out of long-dead colleagues' works and palm them off as their own or who plagiarize a piece introducing it as a new popular song.

Some composers are able to combine the two forms, acting as both a primary and a secondary channel in the same full-length work. Ralph Vaughn Williams did this with his *Fifth Symphony*, combining folk music with his own inspiration.

The realm of music has its own spiritual helpers and archangels, who sing tunefully to all those who concentrate their life's growth via music. Whether one is a secret composer basking in obscurity, a struggling artist who isn't able to sell the fruits of their labor, or a well-established luminary, the spirit helpers channel to all. Many catch the same message and interpret it in their own way. When this happens with the musically successful, several songs that are very much alike may appear on the charts. Each channel, having filtered it through their own personality and intellect, has made something distinct out of it. And, if the songs are timely by Universal standards, all can be hits at the same time.

In the mid-1960s Burt Bachrach was interviewed on the radio. He explained that he and Michael Lerner each had a song on the top forties chart that was appreciably like the other's work. He named a third composer whose similar piece had also climbed into the hit parade but had not done as well as his. He lay the credit for such coincidences at the door of the angels who deliver music to our plane.

At concerts I always watch the singers and musicians to see what type of guide they possess. Oftentimes the musician has a guide for their playing and a guide for their instrument. Holly Near has a sprightly green, miniature figure who dances across the stage as she sings. For a person whose music is about universal love and acceptance, the color of her singing guide is absolutely perfect. George Winston, a secondary channel, has an everpresent entity hovering over the piano as he plays. His guide is far more serious than the kindly musician whose playing he oversees. Classical guitarist Neill Archer Roan has a guide for himself and two for his instrument. He approaches his performances with a prayerful, sensitive attitude. The more attuned to the Source a musician is, the more gratitude they have for the grace to be a public performer, the greater the presence that comes to guide them on their way.

4
MEDICINE SOUNDS

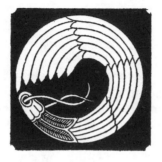

Medicine Sounds

There are many ways the human voice can intercede, altering a situation that appears to be ill fated, enjoining the Universe to be merciful and thereby deliver a favorable outcome. Here we explore a two deeply mystical and powerful singing methods. The first is our own personal Healing Song, with which we balance and realign the health spectrum for ourselves and others. The ultimate vocal expression for personal power and empowering your spiritual nature is your Lifesong.*

The Healing Song and Lifesong are each highly personal, belonging only to the individual through whom they come. Both of these songs operate independently. Each has a place in your life. By carefully following the instructions in each section of this chapter, you will be able to find your personal power songs and sing them successfully, knowing when each is called for under infinite conditions.

You need not be a saint or even nearly perfect to utilize these powerful vocal tools, however, a word of warning: Anything mis-

---

* WARNING: If you skipped the introduction please go back and read it thoroughly before proceeding.

used consciously will boomerang. If you sing the songs with good-will for others, working towards forgiveness and unity, even if you are a bit confused or do the wrong things unintentionally, there'll be no damage. For it is our *intention* that is conveyed in the sounds. Although we might not verbalize our true thoughts, they emanate from our unconscious as we sing, and our own feelings are often purified in the process.

Healing Song

Your Healing Song belongs only to you. It is personal and pub-lic, it heals, comforts, and alters whatever condition you need aid with. You can sing it anytime for anyone. It can heal a child, an adult, a friend, a stranger or a social situation. If any of your relationships become a bit sticky or downright unbearable, your Healing Song can alleviate much of the distress and bring clarity and insight to you so that you can cope better and, perhaps, be more creative about finding solutions to your problems. The Healing Song works on the mental, physical, emotional and spiritual levels of your body/mind.

Your Healing Song has always been with you. You have never been without it, yet you haven't had conscious knowledge of your song. In Western society we ignore the sounds that babies sing. Often little children have a "nonsense" song that is just theirs. In England a rather intuitive Mum I know heard her infant son sing a certain melody repeatedly. She called it his "comfort song". She and his father, both Alexander* teachers, encouraged him to sing it when tired or cranky.

One afternoon the babe, Rupert Egan, and his mother, Sumi Komo, joined me on an outing to a special exhibit at the Tate Gal-lery in London. A museum guard attempting to be humorous said to Rupert, all snuggled against his mother in a baby frontpack, "No singing in the gallery," referring to crying, of course. But eight-month-old Rupert thought the guard meant he couldn't sing his "comfort song". He looked bewildered, almost hurt. This is precisely what most children are told, "Be quiet, suppress your inner experience." Very few parents or teachers realize that the songs of children are often their Healing or Lifesong. Rupert, now an alert pre-schooler,

---

* Alexander, a healing technique for using posture, motion and breathing, to deal with and change unconscious habit patterns.

has continued to comfort himself with his Healing Song. He also sings saga songs about his experiences to integrate them into his life.

When we were children we all had our own songs which often didn't fit our mother-tongue. Most of these songs contain seed sounds that aren't from spoken languages with which we are familiar. Once, when speaking with a middle-aged Pomo Indian woman about Healing Songs, she said, "Yeah, we Indians always get such a laugh when white people sing us a Healing Song in English. They don't come in English."

At Tule Lake Reservation the elders began drumming and singing again after years of separation from their own spiritual practices. The government of the United States, as part of the subjugation of Native Americans, had banned the practice of native religion. When the law was changed, after over eighty years without their own heritage, they began to worship in their ancient spiritual manner again. They couldn't understand the words that were coming through to them even as they sang them. Tribal elders turned to the children four years of age and younger, whose channel to Universal Consciousness is still open. The children explained the words of the "twilight" language. These sounds are called Vocables*.

American Indians aren't the only ones who speak of this twilight language for spiritual activities. In *Women of Wisdom* (published by Routledge and Kegan Paul P/C, 1984), Tsultrim Allione discusses at length what the Tibetans call the language of the *dakini*. "In our culture, which is dominated by the rational, scientific point of view, we tend to think of language in a very limited way. But, mystics and madmen have always maintained that there are other kinds of languages. These are languages which cannot be interpreted or understood by the rational left hemisphere of the brain. The Tibetan lamas speak of a language called 'the secret signs and letters of the dakini (mKha'g ro gSang B ibrDa Yig)'. . . . "

Fundamentalist Christians have a practice called glossalia whereby they receive messages in Anglicized gibberish, which they translate to standard English. In doing so they use too much of the rational mind. It is best to let the mind remain empty and allow the sounds to be whatever they are, without interpretation. In time, left to your own intuition, the seed sounds will let you know their meaning.

Therefore, when you hear your song for the first time and it seems to be nothing more than babble, do not dismiss it. For the

---

*A word or term regarded as a unit of sounds or letters rather than as a unit of meaning.

words, should you receive them immediately, will not be in Chinese, Spanish, Sanskrit or any ancient earthly tongue. They will be in one of a multitude of twilight languages, which seep through the gate that leads from the Realm of Creation to the Physical Realm and vice versa.

Your song is distinct from anyone else's. Some sound like Arabic melodies, others like Hindu or Tibetan chants. The majority sound like American Indian songs. One woman, who taught Sunday School, was astonished to find she had an Israeli-sounding set of musical phrases. A man whose song had great power for him received an atonal, utterly boring set of sounds, which other people said moved them a great deal as he sang.

Commonly the Healing Song has no words in the beginning. Students often report that they have only a single phrase of music. Many get the words to their song as they sing it out-of-doors. Others report that their song has no words whatsoever, and they feel cheated. Occasionally, someone has the words but no tune other than a certain cadence. It is perfectly all right to let it develop as you sing it, for that is the way Universal Guidance delivers your song. The part most familiar to you is the one that arrives first. It is the memory of the higher self that brings it back into focus.

Sometimes the song seems to leave you for awhile only to return later. One woman, thirtyish and intellectually gifted, had taken a series of workshops with me over a two-year period despite her skepticism. Like other members of the class she promptly received her song and went off to sing it alone. But, she was unable to locate her Healing Song after a workshop. Eighteen months later she repeated the Sound Medicine Workshop. This time she took no chances. She recorded it on tape. That is precisely the way to stymie further development of your Healing Song. Taking my advice, she erased it and now has a wonderfully varied song with a strong central refrain.

There are many methods for finding your Healing Song. You can fast and retreat for a week while seeking it. Or you might meditate exclusively for the purpose of hearing it. You can ask for it in your dreams night after night until you recognize and remember it once awakened.

The quickest way for reuniting consciously with your Lifesong and Healing Song is the one I use in my classes. It has successfully delivered these two important personal songs to hundreds of people I've instructed. I drum for ten or fifteen minutes. The song comes through for all but a few skeptical people, who usually say, "Well,

I heard this thing but that couldn't have been my Healing Song so I ignored it and nothing came."

Ordinarily it takes only five to seven minutes of drumming for the most resistant person to tune in to the basic melody of their own Healing Song. From inside the sound of the drum a melodic or haunting song echoes forth. I vary the beat, rhythm, and other factors so the drum will sing out the song of every individual present. I hear the song that belongs to each person and can tell when they have also heard it. Once the drumming introduces the Healing Song, each person puts on their shoes and goes outdoors to sing and dance what they've received.

Frequently, the Healing Song has several sections to it which manifest as you sing it over and over, moving your body to the beat. The words, if they don't arrive at the time you do this exercise, will come after a few weeks of practice singing your song. The more you use it, the wider and deeper it becomes. The only stabilizing element may be the original part the drum gave you, while the rhythm, or the melody or the seed words change during a specific healing.

My own Healing Song begins and ends the same way, but several variations of the middle stanzas may arise during healings. I never know in advance which alteration will manifest as I begin to sing over someone. This form of singing can last five minutes, for more than an hour, or all night long. The song lets you know when to stop. My advice is to let the song be the judge of when the healing is over. It will cease to give you voice or will feel forced when the person or situation being healed has absorbed all they can.

Obviously, I am not present to drum for you. The best way is for you to borrow a drum and experiment until you've found a pattern of striking it that elicits a beat you're comfortable with. Play it until you are satisfied that the beat you have is one you like. A drum takes time to warm up. The inner sound will resonate clearer and fuller as the drum heats under your hand or the drumstick. The best drum for this purpose is one with a natural hide. The plastic ones or those used in bands aren't able to vibrate correctly for the song to sing inside the drum. A dumbek or any open-bottom drum works easily for the novice. If you can't locate that type, a drum with two hide-covered ends will be perfect.

If you have no drum and live within a half-day's drive of the woods or ocean, you can find a hollow log and use your feet to beat out a series of sounds through which your Healing Song comes. You could, in desperation, use a table at home which might produce the necessary resonance to let a song sing through your pounding. Make certain your dwelling is empty of others who mayn't appreciate the enthusiasm manifested by your table drumming.

After drumming or being in trance, your song will begin to be sung for you by your higher consciousness. It won't remain static, so do not hold onto it. Let it become what it will. Do not attempt to write it down to capture it, for the song is a living, breathing energy brought to life as you sing it. It will not be a familiar melody from the radio or a lullaby from your childhood (see Signal Song later in this chapter) and, therefore, will have to adapt to you through repetition.

The best way for this to happen is for you to rise and walk outside, letting the motion of your body act as a receptacle for the essence of your Healing Song. Walk around humming it. Go to an open outdoor space and sing it softly aloud to yourself. When you feel you have your song down sufficiently to remember it, go home (unless you are in a secluded open area) and sing it out loud, sing it with a slow pace, and sing it fast. Allow your song to show you its own range. When you sing it to heal, it will do all these things automatically.

As for your inhibitions about being heard or what reactions might await you, remember this song is under Univeral Guidance. You are not the only one putting energy into it. When the Creator grants you a Healing Song it is meant to heal all who hear it. Sometimes in a healing, another person burns their negativity very quickly upon hearing the Healing Song. Most people's eyes light up when they hear you sing it. It seems vaguely familiar to them, even though it's never been sung for them before.

Will Johnson, an anthropologist and author of *Riding the Ox Home* (Beacon Press 1987), made the following remarks about finding his Healing Song during a workshop I gave in San Diego. "There's something that's been waiting to come out of me for years. I remember church music as a child and all the songs I've ever heard. I can quote you a line from "Shaboom Shaboom," but none of those songs really have a spiritual meaning nor a spiritual application. It's like taking part of the power that's there and giving it a minimal form in which to express itself. And that's what I've gotten out of this experience. My Healing Song came long before we started the drum. It started as soon as you began talking about it. It was there, I just simply couldn't deny it. I didn't know if that was the one or not but it just kept coming out the same. I was also rather diffident about singing it because it's still emerging. All of these sounds, as soon as you hear them and you have the mediation of someone who knows how to use them, begin to come out."

One strong word of warning for musicians. Do not publish your Healing Song or embellish it outside of healing situations. Its power to heal can be spent quickly by doing so. Occasionally, musicians state that their Healing Song is one they wrote long ago, sang for a while, and dropped. One said it was a song she'd written many years before, when she was very unhappy. A Dutch rock musician said he was twelve years old when he first heard the tune in his head as he was walking along the beach. He didn't know it was his Healing Song. He just sang it when he felt depressed or alone. The sound of the sea brought his song to him. He described it as walking in a bell of comfort as you hear your own sound.

Many people who aren't musicians have become reacquainted with the Healing Song they sang privately during times of crisis without knowing it was a very special piece of music, exclusively their own.

Several people in a workshops have asked me about drumming tapes. I have to be honest about the effect of live over canned drumming as the best and surest way to contact your Healing Song. The drumming tapes may induce a trance state, but there is little likelihood that the prerecorded drum will sing your song to you. Better to take the time and effort to find your song by a proven method than to face frustration.

Once you have your song, how you use it and what experiments you do with it are left up to your intuitive creative powers. One man decided to teach it to his friends to sing in a healing circle as a boost to his own recovery.

You can sing your song silently inside after you know it. In airports, supermarkets, at work, at dull parties, while visiting a sick friend, your song is as influential as when sung with a full voice.

One last thing about your Healing Song: if you need it but ignore it, the song will wake you up in the middle of the night by singing itself in a dream.

The Healing Song In Practice

People often ask exactly what happens when I do specialized healings where fasting is part of my preparation. Although every healing is different, this is the general format. Depending upon the severity of the illness and what my guides tell me, I fast for two to four days prior to it. I take a drummer along at dawn or twilight to a very secluded natural setting, which either has a spring or a flowing creek on it. As we walk in I sing my Healing Song. During the healing there'll be some remarkable changes in the Healing Song, revolving around the person who has come for the healing and their mental, emotional, physical, and spiritual condition as revealed by the ceremony. When we walk out, once the healing is finished, I'm usually surrounded by the person's guides who have been bolstering us. I am singing their Healing Song, which has been disclosed to me during the healing ritual. I sing it into them, but not as I do it with the drum. When the drum sings, you get it from the trance state the drumming induces. In this case, the person receives it directly via the energy that was manifested in their behalf by the healing rites.

Outside of ceremonies your Healing Song can enter into your practice on a regular basis. As a general rule, with people who have a long time illness, it's best to use the Healing Song, which somehow touches a nerve-center of Cosmic Consciousness. It reminds them that their life is a gift and their soul is not damaged. It also places them in contact with the highest part of their spiritual being. When someone has a chronic ailment or emotional problem the Healing Song reminds them of their oneness with the Universe.

If they have a longstanding inability to love and be loved, I sing my Healing Song behind their back. I have the person lie face down on the table, placing my hands at the nape of their neck and at the bladder points in the small of their back. This is only to reassure them and distract their attention from the song I am singing under my breath. This breaks down their resistance to being healed as I work out emotions they cannot speak of. Sometimes I pretend to cry behind their back to let out tears they cannot shed. All they feel is my hands bouncing up and down while I am mock crying. Often they'll start to grunt and groan into the floor. Later on, some may talk remorsefully or with relief about secrets they had walled up inside themselves as a way of coping.

Chanting the Healing Song inside your head still works because it's heard on the inner planes. When I feel the client is ready, I say, "I'm going to start singing a little song, not one you know." Or I'll tell them out front "I'm going to sing my Healing Song over you." I can feel ultimate skepticism and all their resistance coming up. Initially I sing it low, and if the helping spirits tell me to sing it louder, I'll sing it louder and louder and louder until it is as loud as it can be for that person and the setting where we are. Other times I'll bring it down, down, down, as softly sung as it takes for that individual to accept it. I might sing it for five minutes, or forty, or as long as it is required. Moments before I'm due to close the song, the client will suddenly say, "My shoulder just popped into place, what are you doing?" Not much, is the answer, I didn't have to manipulate it, or delve into their personal life. The Healing Song removed the emotional, psychological, and spiritual pain they'd allowed to enter their body.

Once I gave a healing in a backyard in the northeast section of Portland, Oregon, in a black neighborhood. I was singing over a man who had heart problems of an emotional nature. My drummer had come with me, and several other people were present. Just as I had cleared the man's heart and he knew he had let go, one of the neighborhood kids started to mimic us and called out the window in a falsetto voice, "We love you." This caused us all to laugh, but especially the man and myself, because we knew he'd released the negativity in his heart at that very moment. The grandchild of a preacher thought he was spoofing us. But it was obvious that the child was under Cosmic guidance.

Lifesong

In sharp contrast to the Healing Song, the Lifesong is extremely private. You can't find it when you want it. Past the time of introduction into the physical plane, the Lifesong isn't readily available. It'll sing itself inside of you when you're in for a dramatic lifechange, require a surge of power, or need to be warned that some momentous and splendid event will arrive shortly. It is a secret.

About twenty years ago, before I became aware of the Lifesong's potential, I went to Scotland and met a young man who was on a personal search. With what I knew then, which was rather insignificant, I sang him my song although I had an inclination not to. He became so inspired he decided to go to a small island off the Isle of Skye to isolate himself. I was innocent and didn't know the rules, luckily there were no untoward consequences. Later I learned that the Lifesong is a secret not to be shared with others and to be used for important transformational experiences.

This is your power song. Sing it aloud when you are certain others aren't around, and in a sacred and respectful manner. If someone else sings it they can steal your power and the gifts reserved for you. As with everything I was ever told was forbidden, I broke the rules once I knew them, to see if it were true. For being so testy with my Lifesong, I paid with two years of hassles. The troubles ceased when I figured out the puzzle of how to restore my Lifesong to me alone. Your own Lifesong is equally personal and must be concealed.

The Lifesong is very special, even sacred. It is unique to each person. I sing it when it lets me; otherwise I cannot get my voice into the essential range. Your song will be totally different from your Healing Song musically as well as in the tremendous energy it raises in your body and auric field when you hear it.

The Lifesong has always been with you, at least as long as your decision to be born. I found a Lifesong in someone very newly arrived on the physical plane. Some years ago I helped Yona Ash with the birth of her son. Through the doppler (fetal stethoscope) I heard a sound like a whale song. It seemed impossible that the sound had come from anything in her system except the baby. I gave the doppler to another birth helper, who looked quizzically at me when she heard it. I listened and heard it again. It was so strange that I discounted it.

After the baby was born, the women who were at the birth wanted to sing a song to welcome him. In a beautiful, sunlit room we sang to him. At the end of our song he had a look of bliss on his face. In return he sang the song I'd heard through the doppler in utero. It was his little whale song, sweeter than that of a whale, more of a human whale singing. The song was awesome, thrilling, and impossible to imitate.

To find your Lifesong, follow the same steps as you have already done to locate your Healing Song. Make certain that a few days have elapsed since you learned your Healing Song. Recapturing the Lifesong requires assistance from me for about twenty-five percent of the students in workshops. You are doing this alone, so be prepared to give it several trials before abandoning the project. One of my translators waited half a year before his Lifesong showed up. He kept trying every few weeks until he succeeded.

If you feel unsteady about looking for your Lifesong, wait until it is nearly dark outside. Light a fire in your fireplace or at a campground where you are alone. As you drum, stare into the fire, The power of the fire and your personal power are related; working with both simultaneously will bring your Lifesong into focus for you. Dance around the fire and sing your Lifesong when it comes to you.

If you have a spirit guide, ask your guide to help you connect with your Lifesong. If you don't know your helping spirits read *Companions in Spirit* by Laeh Maggie Garfield and Jack Grant (Celestial Arts, 1984) and get to know your guides.

Once you hear your Lifesong, hum and sing it to yourself in privacy. A car is an excellent place to do this.

The Lifesong usually is a single line of music or repetition of complex sound variations. Most often it has no words. Seattle architect Jack Martindale's Lifesong is an exception to almost every rule. Instead of vocables it has a strong set of words which arrived when he was moving about to hear his song more fully.

A Lifesong removes negative energies that may cling to you. It brings safety in the face of danger. It empowers protective objects and grants power and energy when you need it. It is the essential ingredient in a successful vision quest.

Once you are familiar with your Lifesong it'll fade away for months until it is time for you to have it again. I've always assumed this is the Creator's way of insuring that the Lifesong won't be abused.

When I came to know my own Lifesong, it sang itself over and over again inside me for half a year until the day I knew what it was and what properties it contained. Then it disappeared until right before an extraordinary event that forever altered my life. My own experience and that of others I've spoken with about the Lifesong is that it heralds new eras your life and provides the power to stay on your lifepath.

The Honor Song

Among the Oglala Sioux there is another type of song which is indicative of the power each person holds. The words are in their Sioux tongue, and contain symbolic and understandable meaning. Newborns are given the song at their naming ceremony by elders in the tribe, who may be close relations of the baby. The song is sung by individuals during dances and spiritual rituals in which they are a central participant. Throughout their lifetime, family members and others will sing that song for them to assist in their recovery from illness. At the death of the person, their Honor Song is sung for the last time to guide them easily to the spirit realm.

Whenever the Honor Song is sung, it confers power and guidance upon its owner. The Oglala Sioux have no Lifesong as described in the previous section.

Among the Northwest Coast Indians, the Lifesong functions as an Honor Song. It is known to the family and friends of the person. This song is learned by an individual during a fast and a vision quest. Should the person find more than one song, the medicine people helping them will also fast and say prayers for many days so that the seeker can distinguish which song is actually the Honor Song/Lifesong.

If you want to locate your Honor Song in the Northwest manner, it is recommended that you undertake a fast of limited duration (eight days maximum) and drink forty-eight ounces (one and a half liters) of spring or distilled water daily. Remember you cannot just fit it in between business and family life. Of necessity, you withdraw from public view and retreat completely.

You must have your own spirit guide since you have no spiritual director helping you with this quest. Select a site far from industrial noises and out of sight of shopping centers, tracts of houses, and civilization in general. Fast for a full day before your departure. The weather should be warm and you must take adequate clothing with you. The body can be very delicate in fasts, becoming chilled in mild rain. It is always hard to warm up again once you lose your body heat. Plan to stay out six days and nights. If your song arrives early in your vision quest, you may leave after you have sung it repeatedly and are accustomed to it. Wait a few hours and sing it again to make certain you have committed it to memory. If your song fails to arrive by the end of the fifth night, leave and return home to rest and recover. You may hold a fast and a vision quest again after a few weeks have elapsed. Pray and bring your most humble self with you.

All of these songs, the Healing Song, the Lifesong, and the Honor Song are meant to be sung with full voice whenever feasible. Part of the process of healing with sounds and songs is to heal yourself of your own inhibitions.

The Signal Song

The Signal Song is a piece of music composed and played by others. Most frequently it is a recorded song, or segment of classical music heard in concerts or on the radio. The first time you hear it, it commands your attention. Later on you may find yourself singing a section of it. The words hold a pointed message for you. Listening to the song as recorded you may notice that the words your mind made for the music weren't exactly the same. Commonly, they aren't even close to the actual words, and the ones you sing may change from time to time. Heeding the words will tell you what to beware of or to activate in your life. The Signal Song you hear on a journey may not be the one you hear while running errands. One woman, an apprentice of mine, hears parts of Vivaldi's *Four Seasons* whenever her life is about to swing into high gear. She knows what time of year the heralded event will occur by whether it's the winter, spring, autumn or summer segment she hears. Another woman hears John Lennon's *"Imagine"* whenever she's provided with a good opportunity. Because it is a very popular song she often hears it being played and sung live while out walking or at parties. Those times are even more apropos for her than when the song is played on the radio.

A young man discovered his clairaudient ability by hearing musical selections while engaged in conversations with other people. The songs related to the plans and problems they were discussing. And, he based his advice or comments on what his inner ear heard, with good results. He too has a Signal Song which tells him to take special note of the moment. It is an upbeat, wordless jazz excerpt. Entering a building for the first time, he recognized its strains coming from the upper floor and assumed correctly that he'd be in a mutually profitable relationship with the person he was about to meet. He is.

You may have more than one Signal Song. Students and clients have reported having one expressly for one class of experience, and another that covers a multitude of situations. They have also verified receiving new Signal Songs periodically. The Signal Song can also be a favorite from childhood that is played by the inner self when you need help. It may be one you whistle or sing mindlessly while working. A longtime client of mine from Idaho died and his family asked me to reach him on the other side of the gate. I tuned in and heard these lines. *"We never stagger we never fall, we sober up on Uncle Ed's call. Everybody loves us here so come on all let's give a cheer——"* Calling his daughter back with the messages he gave me, I casually mentioned the song. Dead silence on the other end of the line, was all I heard, as she choked back tears. Then she said, "You got my father. He always sang and hummed that."

Anyone can have a Signal Song without being aware of its implications. If you hear a song playing over and over in your head, take note. It may be your temporary or permanent Signal Song.

5
VIBRATIONAL SOUND

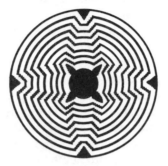

Toning And Overtones

This is an experiential chapter featuring Toning and Overtones, two esoteric healing techniques based on vibrational sound. You are encouraged to use each one of these methods to increase your joy of living. Each mode requires much practice to perfect, therefore do Toning and Overtones frequently. They will energize you and anyone you are healing. Both these practices are ancient and have been incorporated in one form or another into the songs of the major religions. The call to prayer heard five times daily in Moslem cultures is a type of chanting combined with Toning. Amerindians and other native medicine persons use the forms to sing and make sounds corresponding to these techniques. Toning, known by several different names, is also called esoteric sound. Svara is the Sanskrit word used to describe mystic sound or tone. Toning is done in a variety of ways. The one I describe here and teach to my students is the method the Universe delivered to me. It was the technique my teacher, Essie Parrish, sent me out to find, and once I caught it, it became a core part of every healing. Many long months of meditation, discussion, prayers to the Creator, and research went into uncovering these mystical secret sounds.

Each mode is powerful in its own right. *Davening* is a Jewish religious form wherein the observant ones rise and sing their prayers while swaying forward and backward. It is very similiar to Overtones in the quality of sound that's released. It's truly stirring to hear, especially in a room filled with attentive worshippers singing in unison. Most religious buildings have acoustics that support and enhance the Overtones in the music sung and played by parishioners and seminarians who worship or dwell there. Vocal inspiration empowers the people emphasizing their oneness with each other and the Creator.

Toning

Toning is a system of healing that utilizes vowel sounds to alter vibrations in every molecule and cell in the body. Simple to learn and extremely powerful, they fill the atmosphere with sounds that reverberate long after the singer has quit. People find themselves inwardly silent and often unable to speak once the Toning process has been directed at them. When they do return from the mild trance the sound has placed them, in they are quiet, at peace, and restored to balance internally and externally. They say the sounds excite them, release emotional trauma and physical discomfort, at the same time instilling mental unity and spiritual love.

For those of us who aren't familiar with powerful sounds emitted from the voicebox, this may seem quite a lot for one person to bestow upon another. Yet opera buffs go to hear favorite singers not so much for their total performance but for the special notes they are known to hit during stressfully written arias. Most often the operatic devotee awaits the high pitch of the dramatic soprano, who unknowingly strikes a healing chord for the rapt listener. The fan is thereby revitalized by the evening's performance.

When you Tone, it is important to remember that the sounds you are making are for the whole person, not to heal their current health problem. Diseases are not cured due to a specific sound made to destroy them. A cancer will shrink and subside because the individual is regaining their harmonic balance. As this happens the life force of the person can restore vital health.

Often the illnesses people suffer from are caused by chronic stress. We live enveloped by an enormous amount of noise which is beyond our physical and mental ability to cope with. Human beings and other animals respond to loud noises with a rush of hormones being discharged by the body. The hormones help us to gather great speed for flight or to still our bodily sounds and functions until the danger has passed. In our society, ambulances, airplanes, automobiles, vacuum cleaners, and industry destroy our inner harmony with their sonic dissonance. Our bodies have no place to run in crowded offices or schools, nor is that considered an appropriate response to abrupt discordant sounds. To remove the supercharged energy our bodies put out, we are left with exercise at a later time and Toning.

When you Tone for another person, align your energy with theirs. The simpliest way is to either picture in your mind or say their name as you begin. If you don't know them, think of who they are. "Martin's Grandmother" will do nicely as a way to connect energetically; the Source knows who you mean. Usually in a series of seven to ten sounds, you will be able to re-energize the person you are Toning for. Although the number of sounds almost always varies between three and twenty-five, should more Tones be needed, you will feel incomplete and want to continue singing. End on the highest note you can without pushing yourself further than the vocal capacity you have at the moment. Healing in this form is an intuitive process. Altos can sing soprano and basso-profundos often turn into tenors. It works beyond your normal physical limits.

If your sounds are off pitch, it signifies that the person you are Toning for has an extreme imbalance in the chakra(s) where you are working. The Tone will become more centered and harmonious as the healing progresses. The individual will also open to aspects of their conscious awareness that were previously blocked. A spiritual recommitment to life and a recognition of their share of the world's work as a gift rather than a burden often occurs.

Permit the healing energy to overtake you so that you're channeling the healing. Thinking interferes with the flow; you must utilize the part of your mind that senses sans words. You might know, intellectually, that the EEEE sound sung in the right range will cause a bent-under tailbone to pop out, reassuming its normal position. Filled with confidence you make that sound knowing it'll work. You'll be surprised when it doesn't, and you cannot even get that Tone to come out of your mouth properly. Allow the sound to emit spontaneously. Only then are you truly acting as a channel. You don't do it, it does you! When you are not able to get the Tones out at a pitch you believe is correct, drop down an octave or two and clear the lower energies before attempting to re-establish harmonic parity. Let the sound you make be the one that comes naturally and do not force it under any circumstances. Pay little attention to the key. Guidance will lead you to the right key and alter it as often during the healing as necessary. The Tones will change as you do them. Listen carefully, for this is an important part of staying in touch with the progess of a healing.

Once you are Toning there is no need to pause between clients. In absent healings, you can envision person after person as you continue to heal each one. The Toning will become more of a universal sound, reflecting the deepest needs each individual has. All human beings want love and acceptance. The Tones you make will serve to revitalize and balance each individual you intend to heal. In healings where you are there in person, concentrate solely on your client, friend or relative and give it everything you've got.

If you're doing psychological therapy, it is pretty hard to sing over someone. A Licensed Marriage and Family Counsellor or Ph.D. will have to introduce the client to this practice cautiously, explaining what you know about it and giving clear examples. With any kind of touch therapy where you have your hands on someone, you can simply say, "I'm going to do some sounds to help you with your healing." That's a very gentle way to prepare the client. Then whatever Tones you make will relax and comfort them. Often a single healing, when you're there in person, is sufficient to turn the tide from disaster to normality.

Healing Anecdotes

At "Sacred Wallet," the hospital two blocks from my former office, the nurses had become acquainted with my work. Occasionally one or another of them would call me, hustling me in between the last visitor and the doctor's final rounds. A young mother hospitalized for a mysterious form of internal bleeding had been through several surgeries in the past month without success. She was not better and faced another surgical procedure to stem the bleeding. The nurses, who are usually alert to a patient's symptoms, suspected the culprit was rat poisoning. I went to the woman's room after hours. The ward was totally chaotic, because the doctors were in the building and the nurses couldn't have me there without getting fired. Therefore, I had to work quickly. At first I did some sucking doctoring* to rid the body

---

*This is a form of Shamanic healing where the poison in the body is sucked out with or without actually pressing the mouth against the person. The illness is spat out of the healer's mouth.

of the poison, and then Toned for about five minutes. Two days later the now healthy woman was released from the hospital.

A small child had fallen out of her grandmother's automobile, which didn't have safety locks on the back doors. A truck attempted to pass the car, which had slowed down immediately after the two-year-old tumbled out, and it ran over the girl's head. Very shortly afterwards calls began to come in from friends of the grandmother asking for healing, but visiting was restricted to family members. That very day I was giving a class about healing with sound. During the section on Toning I had the class Tone for the child. I also healed her many more times using Toning, as did other people in the community. Within three weeks her head was normal. Her exceptional doctor, an excellent plastic surgeon whose technical skills are far above the ordinary, knew he'd had some help with this child and yet he was astounded by her recovery. He stated that when children whose heads are still growing have massive head injuries, the platelets in the skull don't expand correctly. She would very likely require further surgery as she grew. It's been five years now, and so far none has been necessary.

Inquiries

A student asked if I knew of any cases where Toning did the seemingly impossible. Yes, I knew of a case where a long-time quadriplegic had the use of one arm and her hand partially restored by Toning and crystal healing. People with severe injuries have a second problem, almost everyone around them carries an entrenched belief system that denies the validity of alternative methods of healing. How can they work if medical science can't do anything further? Many times injured people feel it is hopeless, so not only do their physical bodies require healing but their psyches as well. The healer has to transcend their mental barriers in order to be effective.

You can do one other thing for somebody who has been severely damaged whether it's paralysis or a heart attack. Make a tape at least twenty minutes long that tells them they are improving and are now able to use the injured parts of their body. Have the person play it just before they go to sleep or allow themselves to fall asleep listening to it.

As the injured part heals, upgrade the tape so the suggestion is closer and closer to normal functioning. It may take several months or even years for a tape to do its job, but in restoring full range of motion or function persistence counts.

Q. *What do you do when you have a friend in surgery?*

A. Telepathically join them in surgery at the hour your friend is being operated on. The first step is to make some grounding sounds for the medical team so that they are centered and ultra-competent while operating on your friend. Returning your attention to your friend, make some sounds that resonate with them. Tone for them just before the operation takes place, again at the time you think they're midway through, and once it's over. Even if they are anesthetized their emotions will still run high. You'll develop a sixth sense that tells you how much Toning is needed. Once they are out of surgery, it's best to do a few Tones for them every hour, if you can. Remember to Tone for the staff that will be taking care of your friend as well.

Q. *What kind of feedback do you receive when Toning?*

A. It varies. I frequently get fully developed clear pictures that tell me a story. Depending upon how sucessful the rest of the healing has been, I may stop and ask the person for details about what I am seeing. One client, a new mother, had suffered from a persistent bladder infection since the seventh month of pregnancy. She was now nursing her two-month-old and did not wish to continue the antibiotics, which had failed to cure her. I went to her house. It was uninsulated and inadequately heated. We talked about good shelter being an important factor in healing. Following a laying on of hands I began to Tone. I saw a yellow house next to a vacant lot in an old section of town. That image remained from note to note so I stopped and asked her about that house. Her grandparents lived in it. She was eight years old and terrified of being on the second floor. When her grandfather was dying, she refused to go upstairs to say good-bye to him. Everyone in her family was furious with her for failing to see him before he died. That terror turned out to be the actual spiritual/emotional cause of her bladder infection. She planned to take her baby to see her family and was quite fearful that they might disapprove of her once again. After we concluded talking it out I did some Tones to remove the fear.

In another dramatic healing, Pam Lynn Pegg, a childless woman, was referred to me for a cervical cancer termed *carcinoma in situ* CIN III. After about an hour of other types of healing I began to Tone for her. Within a few notes I distinctly saw her as an infant, being hurled across the room head first against the wall. Immediately, I stopped and told her what I'd seen. She could barely believe it. As a baby under one year, she had no recollection of the incident. I named her father as the inflicter and the true source of her cancer. Three months later she sent me a letter saying her mother had verified that she had as an infant been dashed against a wall and wanted to know how she'd ever uncovered the information. It hadn't been her father (he'd only instigated the battering she took by being violent towards his wife, who had flung their daughter against the wall during the argument).

It took more than that one session. We stayed in touch long distance by phone and did other healings when we could get together. Pam Lynn also gathered a supportive network of friends around her while continuing to see Yona Ash, who'd been my apprentice for eight years. Success came after nearly two years of intensive work to heal herself. Pam Lynn has been receiving healthy Pap tests and is now considered cancer free. Today she is alive, healthy, and still has her ability to bear children if she wishes.

Q. *Is it possible to Tone for yourself? How do you know when to Tone for yourself?*

A. Naturally, you'd Tone for yourself if you were ill with a manageable ailment. Remind yourself to also Tone for the vibrational field of your body/mind/psyche or whatever terminology you choose to describe that interlocking system. At times in an imbalanced state, you're all fogged up, but nothing is actually wrong. There can be interference with the delivery of hormones from the endocrine system due to a shrieking auto burglar alarm that went off nearby the day before, convulsing your glandular output. Noises that aren't properly discharged go into to adrenal glands waiting until a buildup causes an actual infirmity such as night blindness or an auto immune dysfunction, e.g. arthritis, allergies, diabetes, or cancer, when triggered by the correlating emotional disunity.

A noteworthy series of experiments have been conducted verifying Toning as healing people rapidly, whether or not they were aware of the Toning.

How To Tone

Each Tone can be most easily sung by holding your mouth as instructed. The postures recommended for your body promote the best Tones. Vowel sounds last the longest, up to fifteen seconds. Consonants at the beginning or end of a Tone fade quickly with the exception of *M* and *N*, which can be held. To make a good quality *MMMM* or *NNNNN* the mouth is closed and the tongue blocks the inside of the mouth. Pursing the lips will increase the volume and remove any tension at the corners of the mouth.

The *MMMMM*, ancient Hindu mystics learned, has an energizing effect on the brain and stimulates the pineal gland, the endocrine gland ruling the third eye (sixth chakra), thereby opening and magnifying intuitive ability. For the singer as well as the person sung for, the sound will vibrate in the head. The middle ear is then able to work better, aiding both sound reception and clairaudience. Intuition is a vital part of our functioning. Since it is still held in wide disrepute by industrialized societies, people are often blocked from their inner knowing and higher consciousness, causing poor communication between the body, mind, and spirit.

The vowel sounds may be sung one at a time: *AAAAA, EEEEE, IIIII, OOOOO, UUUUU, AAAHHH, OEOEOE, ÆÆÆ*; or combined, *OOEEEOO, YAAAA, EEEYAHH*. How the Tones come out of you is the way they are to supposed be. The vowels correspond to the English words, bay # *AAAAA*, tree # *EEEEE*, my # *IIIII*, so # *OOOOO*, shoe # *UUUUU*, ah # *AAAHHH*, bet #*ÆÆÆÆÆ*.There is no English equivalent for the OEOEOE sound. Each sound comes up from your belly where the most natural form of breathing is centered (see the Chapter 12 section on breathing) and flows out, only incidentally gathering tone as it crosses your voicebox and floats out through your mouth. Every sound is multidimensional without effort. There are overtones and undertones to it, and vibrational forces that set every molecule and fiber of the body in motion to reconstitute total balance.

To Tone, stand with your feet about fifteen inches (35 centimeters) apart, knees loose and bendable. Shift your weight from one leg to the other flexing the knees each time you change sides. You will feel suspended above them if your body is properly centered. Pretend there is a cord from the top of your skull to the sky which stretches you and keeps your head floating, tension free, with your neck resting under it. Rotate your pelvis back and forth feeling the motion of your torso. Your entire body must move from the centered pelvis to let the sound issue forth in totally developed notes and rhythms.

If you have difficulty standing fully erect lie down on the floor, feet together, and lift your arms over your head, stretching them towards the wall. Remain in this position for three or four minutes.

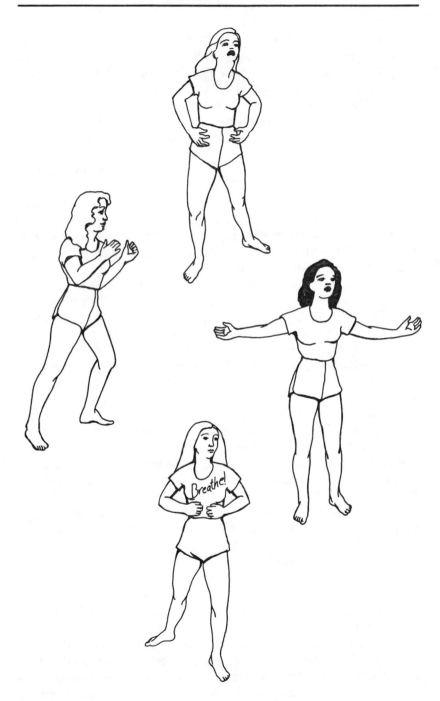

Grab your opposite shoulders with your hands as if to hug yourself, simultaneously lift your upper body off the floor, drop back to the ground, reverse your arms, and repeat. Your back will straighten and you'll notice a release of tension.

Stand up again, head held high, exhale, and bend your right ear to your shoulder as far as it will go without pulling your shoulder up. Do the same on the left side. Hold each side for a slow count of eight without inhaling. Breathe in, exhale and lower your chin to your chest. Keep to a count of eight before taking a breath and only do so when your head is held upright and centered. Let all your air out lifting your head backwards so you can see the wall behind you. Return to center and take a deep breath. Repeat each pose three times. Holding the breath is an important step. One of the goals to aim for is holding the Tone for fifteen unbroken seconds.

You may also do head rolls slowly, ten to the left and ten to the right, to loosen your throat further. Those who exercise regularly are at an advantage in making the sounds work well. A flexible body is as vital as a concentrated quiet mind in effectively working with sound.

Commence breathing in and out without any force. Notice your inhalation and exhalation. Follow your breath; see where it goes in your body. Are there any places your breath does not have access to? Deliberately breathe into those areas. Breathe in through your nose and open your mouth slightly to expel the used air. A bit of soft *shhing* sound may come out with the exhalation. This is normal and beneficial.

Prepare to Tone by taking air into your lower abdomen. Hold your hand there if it helps to establish good habits and concentration. Exhale slowly, feeling the air come up through your entire torso, pass lightly over your voicebox and out of your mouth. Following a few practice breaths add sound to it, letting your full voice show. The tones should be as audible as if they must fill a concert hall.

The *OOOOO* sound is relatively simple, just purse your lips and let the volume out. The *EEEEE* is one of the easiest Tones to hold for a long time. To remedy a lack of sufficient resonance, lift your arms up and out to the side. Have you ever watched opera stars gesticulating with their arms? It's not only part of the acting, it's also to get that note. Arm movements add balance in Toning, especially for an ungrounded person. Pick your head up to increase volume, drawing your chin up just a bit. The same technique will recapture Tone you are losing when you still have breath left inside to sing with. If your voice breaks just continue; it doesn't matter. Go onto the next Tone, noticing your pattern as you sing.

Do movements with the Tone if you feel the inclination or are guided to. Allow the motion to flow from a natural intuitive feeling. These needn't be dramatic or abrupt. Simply shift your weight from one foot to the other bending your knees. They're probably best done slowly and in place like Tai Chi. Incidentally, Tai Chi centers you in your belly, which is where these Tones well up from.

Attune yourself either to your own soul level (higher self) or to another person whom you want to heal. The sounds will come naturally, unforced. Hold the notes for as long as you are able. Before you wobble off key, close your mouth and make an *M* or *N* or any other consonant sound to end. Breathe into your belly again, and repeat the process following any vowel or consonant that comes out of you. Consonants may be at the beginning or the end of the vowel sounds. You may hear them forming in your mind before they come out of your mouth. Permit them to flow out however they come through. Whether it's an R or an H or a J, pay more attention to its quality and fullness than to what it you think ought to be.

An older voice doesn't sound like a younger one. Every so often during Toning instruction some senior citizen will knock me over by letting out Tones the quality of Pavarotti's. Usually, at some point in your sixties your voice undergoes a change. Practice helps retain the flexibility and range of the voice. Choir members or those who sing regularly can go into their late seventies with full vocal ability approximating that of a younger voice.

Overtones

Overtones are resonating multidimensional sounds that originate from a single note. The chanting of Tibetan monks is replete with overtones. Cloistered Catholic monks and nuns sing Gregorian chants, a beautiful, melodic, poetic form of singing containing overtones that echo throughout the chapel and along the corridors of the monastary. The songs serve to clear the mental/emotional planes, thereby permitting greater access to the Source and your own soul.

Overtones is an incorrect and confusing translation from the German word *Obertone*. Uppertones is a clearer and more accurate word for the whole series of higher tones emanating from a musical note.

As an example, when we strike the C-string of a cello or piano, the sound we hear is made up of various tones called partial tones. All the partial tones within a single note are referred to as a compound or complex tone. The lowest partial tone is the fundamental or prime tone. It is the loudest tone of the whole series; therefore we name that string's sound after its prime tone. All the other partial tones are upper partials or Uppertones.

The physical or measurable characteristics of Uppertones are frequency, intensity, and waveform. With special hi-tech devices you can analyze and classify a note, describing the characteristics of its Uppertones. The frequency or number of vibrations of the tone's soundwave per second is measured in hertz; the higher the tone, the bigger its hertz-number.

The intensity or the loudness of a tone is measured in the height or amplitude of its soundwaves; the louder the tone, the greater the amplitude. The form of the soundwave tells you something about the number of overtones that are present in the tone. A complex tone with a lot of overtones shows a widely varied structure while a single tone has a consistent wavy form.

The psychological or aesthetic characteristics that correspond to the physical characteristics are pitch, loudness, and quality. Studying the theory of overtones offers you an opportunity to understand the link between quantity and quality.

Getting back to that C-string, strike it and we hear a note that contains a fundamental tone and an infinite number of uppertones. Each musical instrument has its own sound quality, its own spectrum of overtones. Even if we were well-trained we couldn't hear all of them; overtones higher up in the series surpass our audible limits (16–16,000 hertz). A great proportion of the overtones travel in "silence," as subliminal sound.

The first uppertone has a frequency twice the rate of the fundamental tone; the second overtone has a frequency three times the frequency of its fundamental; the third overtone's frequency is four times, and so on. The hertzian number relationship of overtones has a certain mode that is the same for every fundamental tone. To help you visualize that inner relationship of the partials of a complex tone, compare it with the keys on a piano. Each key on a piano is a complex tone, while a partial is a simple or single tone.

We call the relationship of the hertz-numbers of these partial tones harmonics. Together they create a sound of harmony. In addition to the limits of the audible range, there are limits to our hearing

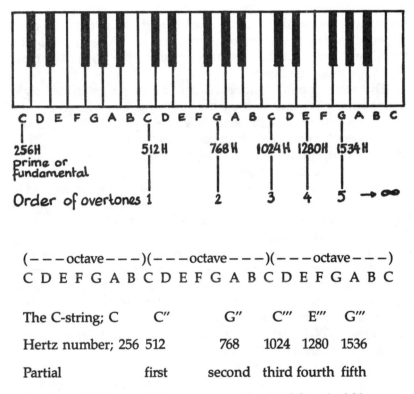

256H
prime or
fundamental

512 H   768 H   1024 H 1280H 1534 H

Order of overtones 1   2   3   4   5 → ∞

(– – – octave – – –)(– – – octave – – –)(– – – octave – – –)
C D E F G A B C D E F G A B C D E F G A B C

The C-string; C	C″	G″	C‴	E‴	G‴
Hertz number; 256	512	768	1024	1280	1536
Partial	first	second	third	fourth	fifth
fundamental tone	first	second	third	fourth	fifth

(– – – – – –Overtones – – – – – –)

discrimination wherein it becomes impossible to hear the separate overtones. Although the measured hertz interval from partial tone to partial tone is equal, the pitch-interval (the height difference of the partials as we hear them) gets smaller and smaller until we cannot hear the difference anymore.

As already mentioned, a complex tone is called after its fundamental tone because of the fact that it is the loudest partial tone of the whole series; the higher in the sequence of the partials, the more its intensity—its audibility in the complex tone's sound— decrease.

Of the separate overtones, the third and fifth overtone we hear best. A major chord in music is a fundamental tone plus its first five overtones played as complex tones. For example, you touch the C, C″, G″, C‴, E‴, and G‴ key on the piano simultaneously. To be able to hear these different complex tones in such a chord requires training. Even more training is required to be able to hear these same overtones in the first C-key alone.

To be able to sing with Overtones you have to relax, shape and train your vocal instrument so that it becomes a willing instrument for our sound. Every natural sound has overtones, it's a matter of creating the right soundbox in your body so that they can resonate .

The physical characteristics of uppertones are frequency, intensity, and wave form. The psychological characteristics are pitch, loudness, and quality. If we strike a middle C, the Mama tone, we will notice that it has children or hertz beyond its own sound. Hertz means vibrations per second. The note you strike is called the fundamental tone. The third and fifth overtones are perceived the best by your ears. Look at the illustration of the piano keys. You can see that the uppertone for middle C becomes G 768 hertz in the third resounding, then C again, followed by E 1280. Therefore, more than one note will be heard in the overtones.

The basic difference between Toning and Overtones is the former aims for higher pitches and the latter seeks the lower vocal ranges. These are harmonic sounds. When people speak of harmonics they mean that something has the same mathematical relationship as the overtones. There are intervals between leaves to a branch, the inner structure of a crystal, the distance between organs in your body all falling within a harmonic range. This is true in buildings made with divine proportions. Paul Horn, the flutist, was leaving for the Great

NOTE: See page 172 to order Sound Medicine cassette.

Pyramid in Egypt hoping to record inside of it, when he received a phone call. The man on the other end informed him that the inside of the Great Pyramid would yield the note A minus 231. Curious as to how his caller knew he asked if the man had played inside of it. "No", replied the mathematician, "I figured it out from the dimensions." Later inside the pyramid Paul Horn discovered his caller had been absolutely correct.

The following vocal exercises will help you to sing Overtones correctly. There are several different methods to help you to harmonize your emotional, physical, spiritual, and mental bodies. Take each of the exercises slowly. You mayn't be able to complete all of them in one session when you are first learning. Begin at the beginning each time and repeat all the steps as they appear below until you have mastered the Overtones. Once you are proficient, you can select any single mode or set of techniques to use at anytime. If you have purchased the tape that is available with this book, you can perform these exercises along with it, otherwise you will have to improvise the sounds as your imagination interprets them from the written page.

1) To begin, lie down on your back and relax. Pay attention to your breath, allowing it to come and go softly streaming in and out. Do this for three to five minutes.

2) Place your hands on your belly and breathe in deeply, pushing the air out through your teeth. Three to five minutes will be enough to remove your normal everyday tension. Then sit up and feel the peacefulness throughout your entire body and mind.

3) Using the deepest, lowest voice range you have the faculty for, without forcing yourself, sing these vowel sounds in sequence: OO-O-A-E-I. Remain mindful of your breathing, letting it come rhythmically and simply. Notice what part of your body the vocals are resounding in. Breathe and sing without effort, creating a unity of breath and voice.

4) Next make certain the sound is coming from your belly the same way you did the Toning in the previous section. Connect the vowels in a graceful stream from one to the other without stopping or inhaling inbetween. Starting with OO, make your mouth small and round. As you reach for the O, keep your mouth round and elongate it to an oval. Retain the length for the vowel A and widen your mouth so that the length and width are nearly the same. The E requires a narrow semi-smile with your slightly arched tongue placed behind your bottom teeth. Moving along to the I, your mouth

becomes broad and fully open. Each time you finish a sequence, return to the beginning and sing the mantra again in the same order. Practice this until you are mindlessly able to perform the sequence.

5) Progressing further, your lips begin to do the work becoming tauter and your diaphragm tenses to produce true Overtones. The voice settles into your head, resonating in it as you chant. Your nostrils feels as if they desire to be pressed together. The sound develops a nasal quality as you drone it. The tongue is rolled backwards, moving minimally back and forth. Your lips make miniature movements to express the OO-O-A-E-I sounds. Continue these sounds until it is completely effortless to remain taunt and yet relaxed while singing. This is called the drumming technique. If you listen to the rhythms of Tibetan monks chanting, you will often hear the same cacophony and an oceanic murmur runnning through it, as you will when a roomful of people chant OO-O-A-E-I.

6) The Bell Rhythm requires that the mouth be opened rather wide. Open and close the glottis, the miniature tongue at the back of your throat, repeating the sounds GING-GANG-GONG-GING-GANG-GONG continuously. You will hear the Overtones most clearly within yourself. Gregorian chanting, once sung daily in Catholic monastaries, most closely approximates the dynamic of this Overtone.

7) The following is the lip-rhythm. MMMMM is the consonant sound made in the front of your mouth between your teeth with your mouth closed. Practice for a moment or two using your lips to pout. Now open your lips slightly for the sounds: MIM-MEM-MAM-MIM-MEM-MAM-MIM-MEM-MAM. Make them by moving your tongue minimally back and forth. The rhythms flow out of that movement. This sound restores your ability to hear in the lower and higher frequency ranges at the same time.

8) When you are finished, lie down again on your back and relax. Breathe in and out, expelling all the air until you are empty inside before taking another inhalation. Rest.

There are numerous quality tapes on the market which very adequately express the Overtones. Listening to these tapes is really relaxing. You might also try singing a duet along with the tapes.

Some recommended ones are:

Stephanie Wolff: Obertone; Micheal Vetter: Missa Universalis, Tambura Priludis, Overtones.

6
SACRED SOUND

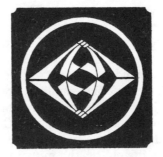

Chanting

Chanting is a vocalized meditation that concentrates all of your attention in the moment. Because chanting is a present time activity, thinking distracts and confuses you thoroughly. Your mind is forced automatically to direct itself to the sounds you utter. Chants utilize the principles of Overtones, Toning and repetition to alter mental, emotional, and spiritual qualities in the individual. Mantras and chants are sung to invoke beneficent aspects including unity with the Creator. They also serve other equally important purposes for maintaining the receptivity and balance necessary for spiritual attainment. Globally, mantras and chants are sung by every religion and sub-sect.

Chanting is done in monasteries, especially those where silence and abstinence are obligatory so that the life force of the renunciates isn't destroyed by lack of vocal exercise. Singing is related to the sexual and artistic/creative channels of physical life. If we are entirely celibate we mayn't be able to let these energies release sufficiently, shutting ourselves off from good health, unless we chant. *Si non copulatus, cantito.*

Secular individuals chant to release psychological and physical energy stagnating in places governed by the fifth chakra and to allow themselves more spontaneity. Improved hearing, better eyesight, sense of smell, taste, and more circumspect speech are the rewards for chanting. Chanting can clean and clear all your chakras, create a relaxed atmosphere, relieve anxiety, remove fears, obliterate negative vibrations, bring mental clarity and inner peace. It can also bring world peace.

Scores of American Indian medicine people chant daily unless they are horrendously ill. Many Native Americans begin every day with a mantra thanking the Creator for the new day they've been given. When Tibetan Rimpoche Chakdud Tulku was very sick, a young monk went to the Tibetan Library to chant from the special books housed there. Those chants recited daily healed the world traveling teacher and physician. Chanting also serves to open the fifth chakra of devotees who repeat the mantras daily. The sounds are seed sounds just the same as Overtones and Toning. They have been formed into words that are given various meanings by translators, none of whom agree exactly, although most of the individual words are names for the Creator. No matter, the mantras still have power and some are used for special purposes with fine results.

Chanting To Clear The Chakras

A very fine chant which uses a separate word for each chakra was discovered by mystics who lived in caves thousands of years ago. They experimented and these sounds came to them via long meditative projects as the correct ones. The word for each chakra is sung nine times, holding the note for as long as the breath lasts. Inhaling deeply, fill your abdomen, rib cage, shoulder girdle, and collarbone with air. You sing the syllable holding the vowel for as long as you can, and then close humming the MMMMM at the end of each word with the exception of the Ah phone. Expel the air first from your collarbone and shoulder area, then from the rib cage and lastly from your abdomen as you sing. Sitting in a balanced pose, the sound lasts longer because it comes out of the hara (chi) center in your pelvic girdle. The positions for maximum energetic flow are tailor fashion (seated on the floor with your knees bent, one foot in front of the other), lotus asana as in yoga, sitting in a comfortable chair, feet firmly on the floor, zazen style on a zafu with your legs folded in front, or standing erect with your feet shoulder width apart. If you are sitting in a manner that blocks the energy, the sound will not be resonant. These postures are recommended for all the chanting and mantras you do.

You do not need to concentrate on the sounds lining up with the chakras. That process is automatic. The sounds themselves cleanse the chakras; all you need to do is observe your feelings, images, and clairaudient messages that arise spontaneously.

LUM	First chakra
VOM	Second chakra
RAM	Third chakra
HUM/EYAM	Fourth chakra
AH/HUM	Fifth chakra
AUM	Sixth chakra
SILENCE	Seventh chakra

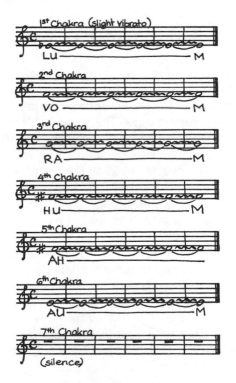

Notice that there are two sounds for the fourth and fifth chakras. Tibetan Buddhists have usually ignored the bodily chakras numbers one to three.

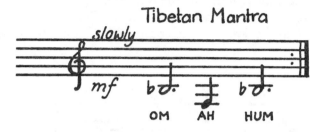

Their well known chakra mantra OM AH HUM is incorporated into a multitude of chants of longer duration, as well as being sung on its own. It functions superbly for aligning the fourth to sixth chakras. Teaching in Western countries the HUM and the AH phones created substantially better inner clarity for the participants than the more traditional Sanskrit ones. The seed sounds EYAM for the heart chakra and HUM for the throat are included here in case you are more attuned to the Hindu form and prefer to sing them when doing chakra cleansing.

Every sound is sung nine times, pausing for a full breath before each one. Rest between the seed words for the next chakra by breathing in and out for a full minute. Sing any note you wish. Do not attempt to restrict the pitch or keep it from going off key. It may become higher as the chakra becomes clearer or will fall octaves as it cleans deeper, less accessible parts of that energy center. Sing it only nine times. If a chakra still feels somewhat unbalanced when you've completed all of them, go back and redo it afterwards, chanting the syllable the full nine times. For the seventh chakra all mystics and religions agree, silence is the correct sound. You cannot keep cars from honking in the street below, or the neighbor from flushing the loo, but maintain your own silence for as long a duration as it took you to sing the sound for a single chakra.

It takes anywhere from twelve to thirty minutes to complete the entire chant, depending upon how long you hold each note and the rest stops in between. Singing it in the car is feasible and it works quite well since it is a private space. You, of course, don't close your eyes while driving irrespective of what song you're singing. Chakra sound meditation isn't likely to make you drowsy. It's effect is total awareness and clarity.

Another chakra cleansing chant is *AH-A-E-O-OO*. *AH* is for the throat chakra, *A* is for the power chakra, *E-*is the root chakra, *O-*the sacral chakra, *OO-* is for the heart chakra. The vowels have a cadance but no formal music. Your sing them without stopping for air. There is no pause between the last sound and the first. It's a continuum, you can chant as long as you want. When you are done, rest and reflect.

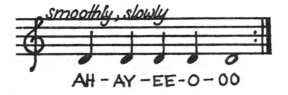

AH - AY -EE-O - OO

Tara's mantra aids you to develop and dispense compassion for all you meet, irrespective of their relative position in life. This mantra sung in rounds of 108 times ends suffering in the lives of the singers.

OM TARE TU TARE

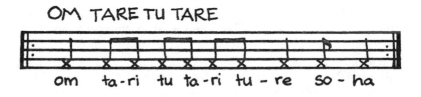

om   ta-ri   tu ta-ri tu - re   so - ha

A very beautiful highly empowering chant credited with originating in several different cultures is presented here. People singing it have had their batteries recharged and are filled with joy afterwards. For men who are accustomed to having words sung in their own gender, it'll feel a bit strange at the beginning. It's a superb practice for experiencing firsthand what language discrimination does to your head. Since all our psyches are composed of both masculine and feminine, it honors our usually under-appreciated powerful, constructive female. Both men and women claim it has a validating effect.

Sing the first two lines of each stanza twice. The name of this chant is:

Daughters Of The Earth.

We are the daughters of the earth.
Born from the place where the sun comes up.   (repeat)
Chorus: She is calling to us. Grandmother is calling to us.

We are the daughters of the sky.
Born from the place where the eagles fly.   (repeat)
Chorus: She is calling to us. Grandmother is calling to us.

We are the daughters of the land.
Born from the place where the tall corn stands.   (repeat)
Chorus: She is calling to us. Grandmother is calling to us.

We are the daughters of the night.
Born from the place where the moon shines bright.   (repeat)
Chorus: She is calling to us. Grandmother is calling to us.

We are the daughters of the sea.
Born from the strength that will always be.   (repeat)
Chorus: She is calling to us. Grandmother is calling to us.

We are the daughters of peace.
Born from the love that will never cease.   (repeat)
Chorus: She is calling to us. Grandmother is calling to us.

We are the daughters of the earth.
Born from the place where the sun comes up.   (repeat)
Chorus: She is calling to us. Grandmother is calling to us.

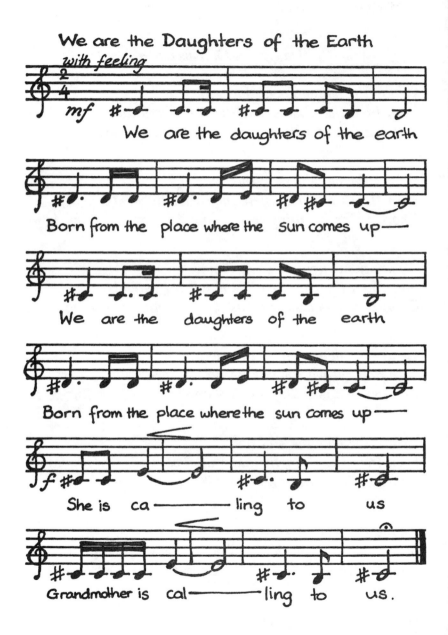

To promote oneness with the higher consciousness, sing the modern mantra written by Shekhinah Mountainwater.

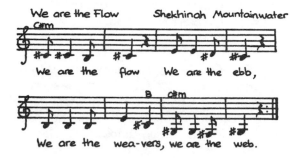

Many families sing mantras over food, sometimes in two or three part harmony, to purify the offering and send thankfulness to the Creator for the bounty given them. A simple mantra that can be repeated before eating, as many times as you like, is Chimes Grace, sung to the tune the bells of Big Ben chime hourly. Amen can be added to your final recitation.

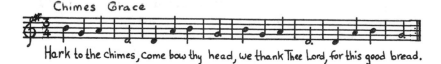

Mantras

Mantra is defined as poetic hymn, prayer, incantation and as the uttering of sacred sounds. Mantras are an integral part of every religious or spiritual ceremony and ritual. In the West we usually refer to our mantras as hymns. Psalms from the Old Testament are mantras, as are some famous toneless prayers that devout Catholics recite. The rosary, a set of fifty small and four large beads (strung ten small one large), is used to say fifty *Hail Marys*, while fingering the small beads. Four *Our Fathers*, another mantra is said in conjunction with the large beads. Protestants, in most sects, sing several hymns while worshiping. Choirs are an important part of Christian liturgical practice. Jews have a multitude of mantras each beginning *Baruch Atah Adonoi, Elehainu, Meloch Ha'olam*, translated as, "Blessed are you the eternal, our God, Ruler of the Universe." These blessings are chanted to deepen their delivery. When sung aloud they go straight to the heart chakra.

Jews also have specific *nusachs* or tonal mantras sung seasonally. Each *nusach* or cantalization contains a melody that must be known to the cantor or singer who conducts the service. More than half the service is sung, in Hebrew, by the cantor with the congregation responding. Witnessing the ritual in all its intensity stirs the mind and heart. Various passages sung from the prayer books* are in different tones according to the cantor who wrote it. Each passage contains psalms, prayers, and praises to God, yet the melody prevails throughout. In the Orthodox sects, the tonal quality is more pronounced than in Conservative, Reform, or Reconstructionist temples.

The *nusachs* follow the seasons, requesting rain in the springtime, becoming lamentations in the fall, before the High Holidays as observant Jews repent their transgressions before God, and another melody for festive holy days as throughout the year. Sabbath services change by the month and have special *nusachs*.

Although it is believed to be more beneficial to utter mantras aloud, they can also be done silently. Many people go around saying their mantra in public without moving their lips. In the days when nuns wore habits you'd see them on public transportation moving their beads, not a muscle in their face changing or showing any sign of the Hail Marys they were reciting.

---

* services assembled from different parts of the Old Testament, with a few from eminent Hebrew scholars like Maimamades.

A well circulated book from a highly-advertised semi-secular Eastern religious movement claims you should always do the very same mantra. If you have no other purpose than to dull the senses, that is true. It is actually best to sing a mantra you like and feels right to you at the time you are chanting it.

Some mantras have been used for so long and held in high repute for thousands of years that they work, if only from the accumulated merit of millions of voices which have sung them. These mantras have been incorporated into current religions that have superceded earlier ones.

One mantra, in circulation for millennia, has the ability to avert physical danger. Singing it for someone who is in potential trouble can stabilize their situation:

Shree Krishna Govinda Hare Murare
Hay Natha Narayana Vasudeva

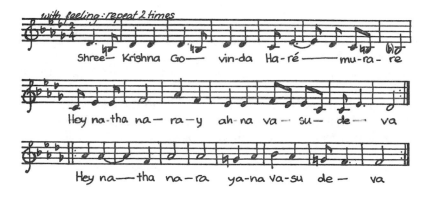

First sing it through twice, then sing the second line twice, then the first again. The chant is then repeated singing the two lines together once, the second line twice, the first line again and so on until you are done. You can sing it for ten minutes or three-quarters of an hour non-stop.

The mantra most effective in dispelling depression is this melodic prayer:

Devakinanda Gopala

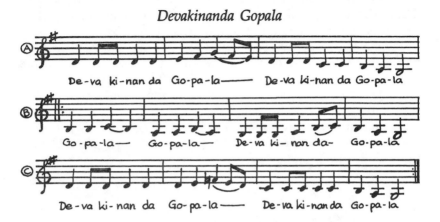

Chant it in this order. Devakinanda Gopala, Devakinanda Gopala, Gopala, Gopala Devakinanda Gopala. Repeat from the beginning. It's tune is lively, lifting the spirits.

States of joyousness are achieved from chanting the Sufi mantra whose words are the same both backwards and forwards. In groups, this chant is accompanied by a circle dance, four steps to the left, four steps to the right, everyone takes four steps into the center, arms uplifted, and four steps back out to the full circle. The dance continues beginning with four steps to the left again. It gets your blood going. Yet the mantra is equally powerful when you are alone. It means peace be with you, be with peace.

Asalaam Aleikhum, Aleikhum Asalaam

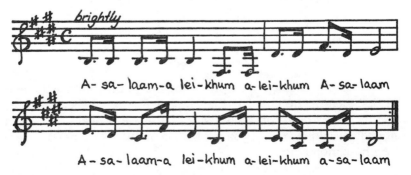

Mantra Madness

Never buy a mantra from anybody or any organization. There's a famous story about a once-popular spiritual group that sold mantras for a $200 initiation fee. With inflation over the years the fee kept rising until some folks paid a thousand dollars for their secret mantra. At a party held by one branch of the sect a few members broke the secrecy, discovering to their embarrassment they'd all been sold a private, specially made set of sounds that was exactly like everyone else's. The revelation spread from one city to another and all told there were only ten "secret" mantras for sale. The question then became, "How much did you pay for your mantra?" Knowledge of the fraud destroyed the sect, which has been slowly rebuilding on the next generation of seekers, each of whom pays for their "secret" power mantra.

Personal Power Mantra Meditation

The personal power mantra meditation and the stories included about it were told to me by Jeanne Etter, founder of Open Adoption Resources. The words or vocables you receive are strictly your own and may arrive in any known language or spiritual tongue not of the earthly plane. Your mantra truly belongs only to you. No money changes hands to have it whispered in your ear. You simply ask the Universe to give you the words and the music, if there is any, which will empower and open you to further spiritual growth.

The instructions are merely to sit in expectant meditation silently awaiting the delivery of your mantra. The first words you hear will be your mantra. Jeanne was disconcerted when her personal mantra sounded like a dish on a Chinese menu. A man in Quaker Meeting sat patiently every day for several weeks without results. One Sunday morning in the Meeting House he was meditating on his power mantra when he heard a child's voice in the garden call "Mommie." He listened and heard it again. "That can't be my mantra," he thought, rejecting it, but he tried it and it was.

With stories like these, I had low expectations for the mantra the Universe might grant me. Anticipating a long wait, I silently did a mantra I already knew, as Jeanne suggested, for preparation. Suddenly I was in a tri-colored visual field with symbolic pictures, each containing instantly discernable personal meaning for me. The voice which delivered the mantra was deep and male, certainly not what I'd been expecting. Kind of word and gentle in tone, He showed total acceptance and approval. The single word He gave me to say is one of the most secret names for God. It was so charged with Universal Light that I immediately went into a state of bliss, remaining that way for seven months, renewing it daily by chanting the name over and over. Mantra meditation turned out to be one of the most powerful experiences of my life. The sound takes me to the place of nonaction where everything is in a perfected state of universal love.

Other people I have shown this method haven't had as dramatic an introduction to their mantra, but all who continue to chant it regularly have extraordinary changes and successes in life. The personal mantra gives a person the courage to be a spiritual warrior.

Ajapa

Ajapa is a silent involuntary form of mantra meditation. It occurs with every breath. Some swami's claim the sound is *Ham* (in breath) *Sa* (out breath): Hamsa. Others believe it is the opposite, and have their followers recite *Soham* when actively reuniting with All That Is. Most Hindu masters teach it so that the faithful will know they are part of the Creator and the Creator is part of them. The exact translation is "I Am That, That I Am." The Chinese call it *Hangsa*. If you hear someone doing this mantra loudly at night you'll call it snoring. Listen, and you'll hear those words Hang ... sa in all the noise.

The way to do the mantra consciously is to say *So* simultaneously with the inhalation and *Ham* on the exhalation, or you may choose to do the opposite. Whichever one you decide, stick to it. Do not switch back and forth from Hangsa, to Soham and Hamsa. You will have ample opportunity to try the various forms in subsequent mantra meditations. Simple as it seems, *Ajapa* requires intense watchfulness. You must constantly be aware of your breath; it will be uneven one time and regular the next. Inhalations and exhalations differ in length. The inhalation mayn't immediately follow an out breath. There will be times when the breath is still.

We are not the only species to emit involuntary mantras. "A cat's purring is like a mantra. They sing it when upset to soothe, when we pet them to admit pleasure. They also sing it when next to another cat being groomed or lying down comfortably," according to Dr.

Michael Fox, veterinarian and author. Anyone who has ever been owned by a cat will agree.

More Mantras

In every workshop students request a mantra to remove destructive thoughts others have sent their way. Tibetan seed sounds comprise this mantra, used from antiquity to banish negativity and send it back to the Source, where it will be positively recycled. The sound *phat* pronounced "fhat" is emphasized, loud, and clipped. It is said ten times forwards and once backwards. You needn't think of anyone to send the bad energy to. This is one time when the Universe will take care of it.

Ah Ka Sa Ma Ra Za Sha Da Ra Sa Ma Ra Ya PHAT! 10 times
PHAT Ya Ra Ma Sa Ra Da Sha Za Ra Ma Sa Ka Ah! once

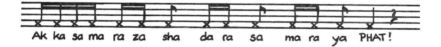

To connect with inner knowing for the highest good of all, sing the next verse over and over, until your mind is beyond the five senses and ordinary reality.

Release your mind, see what you find,
Bring it all home to your people.

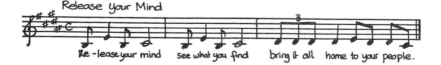

There is a romantic, beautiful, poetic song we sing to babies and young children which retains the capacity to comfort adults who heard it as children. It is sung by mothers in many lands.

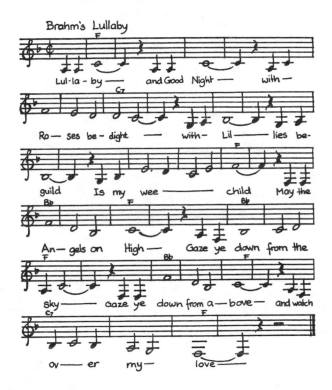

Brahm's Lullaby

English:
Lullaby and Goodnight,
With Roses Bedight,
With Lilies Beguild,
Is My Wee Child,
May the Angels on High,
Gaze Ye Down From The Sky,
Gaze Ye Down From Above,
And, Watch Over My Love.

German:
Guten Abend, gut'Nacht,
mit Rosen bedacht,
mit Näglein besteckt,
Schlüpf unter die Deck:
Morgenfrüh wenn Gott will,
wirst du wieder geweckt
Morgenfrüh wenn Gott will,
wirst du wieder geweckt

Sing Brahms' Lullaby to yourself as many times as you wish in any language. Sit back basking in the peaceful comfort of being well loved.

7
SUBLIMINAL SOUND

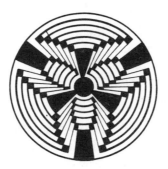

In modern times, industrial pollution in the form of sound is so acute that one can go to the highest mountain in a remote region and still hear the drone of aircraft overhead. We are barely ever free of noise pollution. This is one of our civilization's most disturbing factors.

In our present lives, we are stuck dealing with sound pollution, irrespective of our beliefs about quiet as an important healing mechanism. People living near airports have an illness rate in excess of 20 percent higher than an equivalent population whose homes are not in the vicinity of constant air traffic. Yet airports continue to expand in residential neighborhoods. Airlines may alter flight patterns but that does little to alleviate the noise emissions.

Other industries are equally capable of ignoring sound pollution, as they have other health hazards they thrust upon us by contaminating the water and air. Someday we will run out of fossil fuels and need to rely on other sources of energy. Perhaps scientists and mystics will work on this project cooperatively, so that we can successfully master the art of propelling and warming ourselves with silent power generated by quartz crystals, similar to those used in watches and computers.

Everyone experiences noise pollution but few dare to do much about it. Occasionally, we ask a neighbor to turn down the radio or to postpone using that most irritating of yard items, the power mower. Statistics compiled by the National Institute for Occupational Safety and Health show that prolonged exposure to sounds above 85 decibels can inflict permanent loss of hearing. Short bursts of the same noises can temporarily affect hearing from a distance of five feet (1.5 meters). Some typical loud sounds and their decibel level are listed below:

jet plane takeoff	140
handgun fire	125
pneumatic drill	116
rock band	110
siren	105

We stayed with some Swiss friends whose home was bordered by railway transformers with a constant high voltage buzz. Although we arrived feeling gleeful and rested, after a night of listening to that sound in our sleep, we were tense and uneasy. The second day we noticed that it disturbed our concentration during yoga. Less noticeable yet similarly distressing were the sounds of traffic passing within a few meters of their house. The sound of cars and trucks diminished during off-peak hours and was seldom heard after dark. But the drone of the high tension wires pierced the double-thick glass windows and the shutters that cover them by night. Our friend suffered from severe family problems. This interfered with her children's schooling and contributed to the nervousness of everyone in the household. As a child in New York City, I noticed the same kind of jangled energy in the homes of neighbors who lived alongside the elevated trains.

Electric transformers on poles near homes unsettle the normal human frequency output, making residents ill and giving them headaches and other nervous upsets. In Seattle, during the warm months, crows deliberately bang their beaks against noisily buzzing transformers until they are electrocuted, blowing the local circuits. City Light calls these frequent power outages Crowbituaries. The crows are dying to tell us to bury those wires that mutilate the landscape and cause mental and physical harm.

It's easy to name the various irritating and injurious clamor we are subjected to, indoors and out, in city and country. Refrigerators drone noisily away, sucking the creative energy out of the house members. A Swiss company, Siber, makes silently run refrigerators, and there's no reason why American manufacturers cannot show the same concern for the health of their customers. Vacuum cleaners scream clean, tearing up the nervous system of anyone within hearing range. Commercial leaf sweepers are extremely destructive to the vibrational field that holds our cells together and have an injurious range of several blocks. Helicopters project violent noise over many miles. Jackhammers, auto traffic, diesel engines, sirens, whistles, and buzzers create a cacophony that robs us of our hearing, invades our privacy, and destroys our equilibrium and our health.

The trouble with shutting down our sense of hearing in order to protect our sanity is that we usually forget to turn it back on again. Over time, the ability to hear anything within that frequency range is lost. When city people who have grown used to the electronic and mechanized sounds in their midst find themselves in the country, they often experience difficulty sleeping because the relative silence is so overwhelming. At the same time they are distressed by the unfamiliar animal cries of owls and coyotes, the buzzing of crickets and katydids or the croaking of frogs.

In other nations there are efforts to reconcile the need for peaceful surroundings and the noise of modern life. The Japanese garden, with its running waterfall or fountains, is one very overcrowded nation's way of dealing with noise pollution. Many European homes have double thick glass on the windows for insulation against the severe cold; however, they also serve as a barrier, when closed, against street noises, providing privacy and a rare commodity, silence.

Albert Einstein was an amazingly creative channel. When he died, they took his brain apart and found that it's volume was a bit less than that of the average sized male brain. Einstein was able to tune into that still, small, inner voice, which is connected to all the knowledge in the universe. The brain has nothing to do with this type of knowing; it is the mind that taps into the Source. Einstein used his unique mental link with the cosmos to tune into scientific laws of the universe. It is very doubtful that anyone could achieve what he did amid the plethora of noise that makes up the modern household.

Radio, especially AM with its senseless barrage of commercials and repetitious music, kills creative genius in the young, particularly the very young. The persistent commercial interruptions and the instant change of topic circumvent the natural development of long attention spans and interferes with later ability to meditate.

Many people become addicted to the discjockey and television personalities as substitutes for human contact. In fear of silence, they become hooked on external noise. Although they may want to develop spiritually, they are unwilling to dump the tapedeck from their car. Additionally they flick on radio or television first thing in the morning, thus destroying any dreamtime connection they may have had with their higher self and also precluding healthy communication with the people they live with.

Part of the problem of addictive radio listening and TV watching is that the content is so abysmal. Norman Corwin, author of *Trivializing America: The Triumph of Mediocrity* (Lyle Stewart, 1986), says, "In entertainment and in literature, there is a deliberate aim taken at a particular audience. An audience whose tastes are not high, and an audience that ranges from passive to voyeuristic, to one that is hungry for kicks, for titillation. That explains the success of the formula novel, the success of many television programs and films too."

But the content of programming and commercials is only one dimension of the problem. The greatest negative element is the frequency of the barely audible palpitations in the visual transmission, which cannot be dealt with except by strictly limiting your weekly viewing to under seven hours. This is about all your system can process effectively without damage.

As an experiment remove the TV from your home for six months. Place it in the closet or in a back corner unplugged. Do not watch it at friends' homes or in public places. Then, as a reward, view a single special program. For a day or two afterwards you are likely to experience nervousness, insomnia, or unexplained anxiety. The frequencies emanating from the TV tube are the cause of your misery since they are not compatible with emotional and mental harmony, nor healthy spiritual development.

Vibrationally European television is preferable to the U.S and Canadian versions. Their PAL system generates 625 lines per picture, which is less discombobulating to the human body/mind than ours with a two image overlay of about 250 lines per image. Our sets, depending upon the make and model, can only handle something between 400-450 lines per picture. Your mind has to account for the difference. Another factor makes European TV easier on your psysche: commercials are confined to certain pre-program times. Therefore, shows aren't cut into segments, nor are movies interrupted for an extraneous word from your sponsor.

Before the age of seven, children can cultivate important openings to the inner light. Once the access route has been created, the teenage years spent seeking conformity and acceptance will not destroy it. In the quieter context of human voices, good music of all types, and time spent in out in nature or in large open parks like Golden Gate in San Francisco or Central Park in New York, access to the Source is cultivated.

Parents must set limits on radio and stereo listening, insisting on low volume and the use of headphones, and enforcing a ban on electronic activity during dinner hour. If young children must watch TV at all, their viewing time should be held to a daily maximum of one hour of carefully selected, nonviolent programming. The limits themselves must be limited, since it is best to provide a welcoming atmosphere for our children and their friends. But as they grow older you can also tell them up front that loud raucous sounds destroy the ability of the conscious mind to contact the subconscious mind for the purpose of information, understanding, or prophecy.

For your own sake, you can protect your third chakra—the chakra that is most likely to be out of kilter from urban and suburban din. One way to do this is to wear a silk shield.

Purchase several yards of silk in a color you respond well to. (For information on appropriate color see Companions in Spirit, Chapters 2 and 12). Wind the silk around your waist and abdomen a few times and fasten it . A silk winding will afford you much relief from noise and subtle vibrational influences. During his surgery internship, a friend of mine made a special band of white silk to wear against his body while at the hospital. He quilted the band with cotton padding in the center and wore the silk next to his skin and facing outward towards his clothing. The width was one foot (30 centimeters) and the length sufficient to pass around his midsection and be fastened with Velcro. (See illustration, following page.)

Memories

Sound, like smell, has the ability to evoke vivid memories of what you heard and felt when you were young or in a particular place. There are generational memories linked to certain sounds as well as personal ones. Familiar sounds and ones that inspired or otherwise influenced us take an integral part of us with them when they disappear from our lives. In early childhood I lived a block away

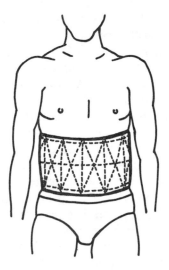

from the elevated trains far enough not to be disturbed by the electronic hum of transformers. The whine of the trains comforted and reassured me in my bed at night, once the noise of the day had waned.

One sound that has nearly disappeared from modern life is that of the steam locomotive. Recordings of steam locomotives winding through the mountains, their haunting whistles bellowing, have the power to bring you right back to that moment when your ears first heard the mournful freedom cry of a train chugging through the countryside. In Basel, Switzerland, I played sounds recorded out of doors for a large group of people whose ages varied from the early twenties to well past retirement. North American birds singing in counterpoint at eventide were not familiar to them and elicited little response other than curiosity. But one sound brought joy to the hearts of all those over forty. Although European tracks don't go clickity-clack like ours, the toot and then the charming whistle of the steam locomotive caused happy memories to surface and beatific looks to erase the lines of tension from their faces. No doubt they went back in time to when they were young and steam locomotives dominated travel. Younger persons listening to the same sound only expressed interest and a bit of mystification as to what had so moved the older ones.

Sounds recreate for us time out of mind or times lost to conscious awareness. We all have memories of sounds no longer heard: horsedrawn carts in the streets below, the special bell the iceman used to inform the neighborhood of his arrival, the jingle the ice cream truck played while you and your friends lined up, change in hand, to buy a cone or popsicle on a hot summer's day, the clinking of bottles as the milkwagon driver went from house to house, the raspy swoosh of coal pouring down the chute into the cellar and the scrape of the oversized shovel on the cement as the last of the coal was cleared from the sidewalk, the used fabric dealer shouting, "I cash clothes," as he rode by with his horse and wagon.

Other evocative sounds that we still encounter today are the twelve o'clock whistle, fire engines, police sirens, school buzzers, church bells that play a certain tune to call their parishioners to worship, excited voices of children at recess or after school, whistles and catcalls at a sandlot ballgame, adult conversation echoing up the canyon walls in cities, the kid next door learning to play the tuba.

There are sounds which elicit negative responses cats territorially yowling on the back fence, screams of pain or anguish, shouting families fighting, the screech of brakes followed by the sound of glass breaking, the roar of a chainsaw viciously attacking a tree, and the great thud of the tree as it hits the forest floor. Motorcycles make a pleasant sounding noise for aficionados and a foul racket for noncyclists. Some people cry when they hear marching bands! Firecrackers make some jumpy while others are thrilled to laughter from the same stimulus. There are people who become excited with anticipation of a good time when hearing the multitude of sounds that make up a carnival. Others are irritated by the same auditory stimulus. This variety of response, even when a sound is loud or raucous, is linked to quality of memory.

Subliminal Sound

The world we live in is one long vibration emanating out of silence. All inanimate objects and things in nature, plants, rocks, and living beings, transmit a vibration that characteristic of their kind. A mollusk vibrates at a rate that lets its predators know it is a mollusk. It has no method of escaping recognition. To evade enemies, a beaver swims underwater quietly, heading for its lodge. It lies low, quelling its normal electromagnetic output. Soldiers and criminals do the same to avoid detection.

In crowds we often make ourselves invisible by modifying our energetic emissions. It's a skill anyone can perfect consciously. Changing your energy waves so others won't be able to identify you is accomplished by altering your thinking. First you cut ties with your personality. This makes you appear to be a human being other than the one you usually present. If you need a little disguising, either wear a wig with your usual clothing or dress in colors you aren't accustomed to. Wear glasses if you are clear sighted and contact lenses if you normally appear in spectacles. Any one or a combination of these will trigger internal mechanisms that change your vibration. If someone looks at you as if they know you, gaze past them; failure to acknowledge or convey recognition is further camouflage.

It is not our looks that let others know it's us. Twenty years ago, the aged German mother of a friend was entertaining our family at her home in Hanau. She often lacked company and was delighted to go many places with us. For one such outing, we went to a town some miles away where there was a famous art gallery. She and I were totally immersed in a picture, when out of the corner of her eye she spotted her finishing school teacher whom she had not seen since girlhood, over sixty years previously. For a while she watched and speculated whether or not this was her former teacher. Leaving my side, she timidly approached her. I witnessed a surprised and elated reunion.

Surely my friend did not recognize her teacher visually. It is not our pearly white teeth, our hair coloring, or our vigorous walk which lasts until old age, nor is it our weight or body build. All of these aspects change along with our faces. What remains the same throughout our lifetime, except when we're mentally afflicted or desperately ill, is the energetic rate at which we vibrate.

Hair

As a student in high school, I bent over the tub and washed my waist length hair every morning before school. The ritual left me clean, clear, and balanced, ready for the new day. Inner knowing told me to do it.

Today scientists confirm that every strand of hair carries vibrations in it. Hair contains the memories of life experience. When people cut their hair, they are excising the intense vibrational recall of that time in their lives. Hair eighteen inches long carries far more with it than three inch hair. Someone who shaves their entire head or, as in current fashion, part of the head, is trying to radically expunge the majority of their memories in an attempt to begin afresh in the present moment.

The military and some religious groups enforce baldheadness to diminish individual identity and the sensory mechanism that hair provides. Other religions want their members to wear long, long hair for in addition to providing a memory bank, hair is a sensing device bringing in telepathic and precognitive information. Remember the story of Samson and Delilah? He had the power in his hair.

To keep long hair clear of unwanted energetic data, wash it frequently, especially when you've been in crowds, airplanes, or hospitals, or when you have witnessed or participated in an argument.

Ultrasound

Waves of energy below the audible range of the human ear are termed infrasonic; those above our hearing range are called ultrasonic. Ultrasound has a wide range of industrial applications such as detecting flaws in solid materials. It is also used in the medical field for destruction of micro-organisms. Sonar, an underwater ultrasonic device, helps to determine the bulk and position of immersed objects.

Ultrasound has brought tremendous advances in surgical procedures, making the invasive techniques of cutting and sewing obsolete. In destroying cataracts, kidney stones, gall stones, and some forms of tumors, it offers a splendid alternative to the trauma of surgical incision and the obligatory convalescence therefrom.

When used on healthy and unsuspecting fetuses, it can be distressing and dangerous. Annemiek Cuppen, an internationally respected Dutch midwife, reports that one minute of diagnostic time with the fetal doppler (fetal stethoscope) is as hazardous as half an hour of the sonar scan. Sonar is intermittent sound while the fetodoppler (doptone) is continuous sound. Most energy is expanding but the doptone is energetically deadening and contracting. "Babies," she noticed, "attempt to move away from the sound." She has felt some of them jump up from sound emitted by the instrument. To best illustrate what the fetus feels, the equivalent sensation is sudden numbness.

Nan Koehler, an active California midwife, says, "Routine ultra-sound in early pregnancy shows many more twins than people thought. Most do not reach maturity and are reabsorbed by the mother's body before birth." Ms. Koehler does use the doptone briefly at nine or ten weeks gestation, because it helps the mother bond with her developing baby. She also uses it for a few seconds at a time during the second stage of labor when the baby is behind the pubic bone and she cannot hear the heartbeat with an ordinary feto-scope. She too affirmed, however, that babies try to turn away from the high frequency sound. She therefore prefers to use it minimally.

Midwives in Western Europe have banded together to educate expectant parents, and those who hope to be parents, to the dangers of ultrasound. As it stands now, German insurance companies will not pay for hospital and doctor services for any woman who fails to have a sonargram at fourteen weeks and again near term. Neither is needed for a healthy mother-to-be if she is under thirty-five years of age. The purpose of the first examination to ascertain whether the mother is actually as pregnant as she claims, is merely to satisfy doctor curiosity. Because little is known about the negative effect ultrasound has on the development of the unborn, it should be avoided.

Obstetric medicine in pregnancy is still primitive. Women delivering forty years ago weren't warned against the ravages of cigarette smoke on the lung development or the birthweight of their babies. Twenty years ago, doctors insisted that moderate alcohol consumption by the mother was no problem for an unborn child; we now know that alcohol can cause birth defects. Annemiek Cuppen reminds us that, about 75 years ago X-rays were routinely done on pregnant women for the same reasons doctors are using ultrasound today. Only when adult men and women began dying in large numbers from leukemia was it belatedly discovered that X-raying fetuses has a potentially fatal delayed effect. To this day, physicians induce delivery and perform Caesarean sections for the flimsiest of excuses, yet people whose birth was forced have revealed the psychological distress carried on throughout their childhood and into their adult years. Only now are these cold, interfering methods beginning to be reassessed by parents, psychologists and natural-childbirth advocates.

Technological gimmicks are no substitute for adequate experience, commitment to normal childbirth, and good intuition. Just prior to a birth, a spiritually well-trained person can mentally enter the uterus and see the condition and position of the infant. Ultrasound dopplers left on throughout delivery only aggravate the birth trauma. In many cases they have caused the baby sufficient difficulty so that surgical delivery became "necessary" as a result of the equipment itself.

The Inner Sounds Or Nadas

Until a few years ago any self-respecting scientist would have denied that the ear broadcasts reference sounds. It was considered only to occur as a pathological disorder called tinnitus wherein persons afflicted with the condition heard buzzing, music, ringing, motors, and other disturbing audible rumblings inside their head or ears. The sounds are loud to the sufferer and when another person places their own ear next to tinnitus victims they can hear a whistling sound. For years medical researchers didn't think of listening for any sounds emanating from normal hearing persons. However, some British researchers decided to place microphones inside the ear canal and were rewarded by finding sound issuing from inside the ear.

While medical researchers debate whether these sounds are produced by the cochlea, or hairs of the sensory cells, they also are mystified as to what they are and why they occur. Mystics in many secret societies and in Hinduism as it is commonly practiced, have known from time immemorial that these are messages from the higher self indicating a level of development the individual must pay attention to. The Sanskrit term for the phenomena is *nada*, or inner sound. Yoga practitioners and meditators seek the inner sound listening to it to aid their spiritual practice.

There are several methods of doing this. One spiritual group that teaches correspondence courses sells its members a special sounding board to magnify the nada. The board is placed across the knees, you prop your elbows upon it while your fingers press against each ear. The more common method is to lie or sit in a comfortable position and place your index fingers up against the little flap that protects your ear canal. Squeeze the flap downward until it entirely covers the ear canal. Keep applying firm pressure from your forefingers against your ears. At first you will hear blood pumping. As that sound fades the true inner sound will emerge. It may become louder and softer or change pace. Do not try to capture it in an appealing form, just listen to it as it ebbs and flows or percusses, noting any rhythm and melody. Often one sound will suddenly end and a new one enter. Allow yourself without prejudice to hear that sound fully. Sometimes they alternate, at other times they supersede one another. Many people hear only one sound for an entire lifetime.

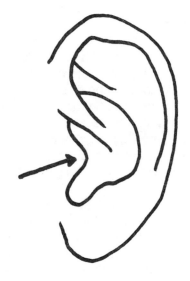

The nadas are related to the chakras and whether you hear buzzing, the wind, or a choir of angels depends on the energy you are mastering at the time. This is your nada and you share it with no one, although others may also hear the ocean as their inner sound. The intensity, volume, intonation, cadence, and frequency are totally idiosyncratic. Nadas are an indication of awakened kundalini energy rising from one rotating wheel of energy to another along the route of the seven main body chakra centers. The sounds and the chakras they denote are listed on the following page.

The practice of listening to the nadas is best done daily. It is particularly fruitful following exercise, meditation or any other spiritual discipline. At times, you spontaneously begin to hear the nada for brief periods during the day. For those whose sound is pleasant there

motors, insects and other buzzing sounds, crickets, electronic sounds	Root chakra
ringing in the ears, running or flowing water, or a waterfall	Sacral chakra
flute	Solar chakra
singing, bells, conch shell, choir of angels, ram's horn	Heart chakra
wind, ocean	Throat chakra
aum sung from the heart	Brow chakra (third eye)
silence	Crown chakra

is seldom any disturbance. If your sound is distressing, when not being sought after, lie down in your own bed if possible, or anywhere you will be at ease for a prolonged period of time, close your eyes and cover your ears just as you would during a meditation on the nada. Readjust your blankets so that you are thoroughly comfortable then lie still, letting the sound roll over you. If it is a motor sound, ringing, or buzzing, it'll become fainter and fainter finally becoming inaudible. Give yourself time. The lifting of loud inner sound may take as long as an hour to remove but then it mayn't reappear for a considerable duration. When the sound is gone, rest for a few more minutes and let yourself relax completely. You will feel renewed and able to tackle anything.

Another remedy for tinnitus is to perform the exercises utilizing the MMM and NNN sounds as instructed in Vibrational Sound, Chapter 5 of this book. Combining both methods regularly will subdue the unwelcomed invasion of persistent nada sounds within your hearing range.

Sometimes a sound that invades your conscious mind is one related to the chakra you are currently exploring and then the nada is a blessing. Distant bells or far off singing often send people to the dentist to explore the possibility that their teeth are transmitting radio programs. While this can happen, before you spend the money looking for an external cure, listen carefully to the sound and hear what it offers you. Listening to it for a quarter of an hour per day may be all it takes to let the spiritual aspect of the nada through. Then you might not hear it except when you are consciously seeking it.

A woman came to me suffering from tinnitus. She thought she wouldn't live another year with that loud buzzing noise, which occurred in only one ear. Her doctor thought he could alleviate it by cutting the nerves which would make her deaf on one side. She decided against that course of treatment. I sat patiently while she unfolded her life story. Though her children were grown and married, they relied on her for everything. Her parents did likewise. Due to their great age she cooked for them and arranged all their outings. She was a devoted daughter. The fatal flaw was that she was angry with her parents and felt obligated to them. She neither liked them as people nor loved them as parents. Added to this she had an exceptionally self-centered husband with whom she was in business . She worked a full day and spent her lunch hours, breaks, and evenings taking care of her family. I told her the buzzing in her ear was a warning to slow down. Unfortunately, she was so driven by guilt that she couldn't stop taking care of others to concentrate on her own health. Shortly thereafter she was hospitalized for exhaustion, totally curtailing her activities and increasing her anxiety about abandoning her family. Her tension and guilt kept the second chakra nada audible. Yet it was a signal of rising kundalini energy which could have been positively used, to increase her own power and vital life force.

A professional man who was often overextended found himself with attacks of tinnitus. He noticed that if he had his secretary hold all his calls for half and hour and placed his head on the desk to rest, the unwelcomed motor sound playing inside his head would fade completely, and he wouldn't be bothered for the remainder of the day. If he ignored the warning signal, it would plague him far into the night, destroying his sleep.

Ringing in the ears can be a message from the higher self trying desperately to get through to you. Stop and permit it to come not by pushing the sound out, but by breathing slowly and rhythmically until you find the information. Usually it is some advise to go more gently with yourself. The stress of late 20th century life leaves us little personal time, and the syndrome of business robs us of the opportunity to listen to the still small voice within, our direct contact with the Creator.

8
COLOR AND SOUND

There is color inside every sound and sound inside of every color. We actually hear color. The inner sound carried by the colors within our eye's range of perception is greater than the number of octaves our outer ears are capable of hearing. There are colors beyond our visionary power in the waking state which come alive in dreams and meditation.

Bring a color you like into your bedroom with new sheets or wallpaper and even in the dark you will sleep soundly because it comforts you. Paint a wall a color you do not like or one which jars your senses and your sleep will become fitful and filled with disturbing dreams.

There are people for whom sound is greater than any other sensory experience: musicologists, musicians, and the blind.

Blind people report seeing colors in people's voices and energy fields. Hearing impaired people often describe the sound they are hearing emitted by flowers, plants, stones, and human beings in bands of color. These color bands of sound vary in size, density, opaqueness, translucency, flow, rapidity, and faintness.

In my student years one of the younger women in our apartment building, blind since birth, described colors she felt as being warm or cool, fat or thin, full, wavering, empty, quiet, loud, picrc-ing, and jumpy. She said they sounded melodic or discordant. I became fascinated with her way of seeing one morning when she asked me to describe the color I was wearing since it was so peace-ful. My outfit was a moderate blue with a complimentary green woven belt. My neighbor could tell a patterned shirt with a vari-ety of colors apart from a simple two color white on green or one with subtle stripes. This was at the height of the hippie era when outrageously wild colors jarred the eye and the psyche. Her sensi-tivity to the sound wave of a color never ceased to amaze me.

In Zen Buddhism the test of an initiate in the Pure Land sect is to see the color in sound and the sound in color. They have a koan for this phenomena.

The hue of the purple robe by the ear,
And the sound of one hand by the eye
To be perceived.

It can take three years to master the sound in color and the color in sound if the meditator takes no wrong turns. Otherwise ten or twenty years can pass before the internal sound of color becomes audient.

Kannon Kan literally means "to see" and *on* means "sound." *The Bodhisattva Kannon,* or *Kanzeon,* is thus associated with what Soyen Shaku call "the seeing of the world-sound," that is, the compas-sionate hearing of all sounds sent out by sentient beings in appeal and desperation. *The Kannon Gyo,* or *Kannon Sutra,* is the twenty-fifth chapter of the Lotus Sutra, and is chanted quite frequently in Japan. Kanzeon is known in Sanskrit as *Avalokitesvara.*

This is the basic principle behind color healing. It is the inter-nal vibrational sound the hue sends forth that heals.

Color healing has been extensively studied and systems that work are known. Yet the systems don't often agree. One may claim miraculous cures from burns using green and another says orange works. In fact they both do. Orange takes away the swelling and green causes rapid regrowth of skin and other tissues. A third sys-tem says to use red with burns because fire fights fire. That one works in some cases. Yet I find drinking water infused with blue light to work better than red to soothe and heal chemical burns.

Colored Water

To make color infused water obtain one liter (quart) jars in clear true colors. Pour pure spring water into the jar and allow it to sit at least eight hours in the window. It does not matter whether the day is cloudy or sunny. Cover the top with a piece of paper or unscrewed-down lid. This is only to prevent insects and debris from contaminating the water.

The water will look like regular water. Nevertheless, purple-infused water will taste like fungus and lemon-colored water will taste citrusy. Drink an eight-ounce glass of water charged with the color you require. You may sip as much as you have on hand. It is not necessary to leave the water in the colored bottle once it has been permeated by the color. Pour it out and keep it in a clean thermos that has not been used for coffee or tea. Refill the jar with spring water to prepare another treatment or to use as needed.

Color lamp

Build a box of wood or make a tube that can act as a shade for a 500-watt bulb. In the front of either one, build a slit panel so that colored glass or gels can be placed firmly in front of the light. Your client lies down under the light and remains there for one hour.

Chromotherapy

Yona Ash, one of my graduate apprentices familiar with my methods for color meditation, flowers, and foods, came to me regarding an older couple ready to retire who had devoted their lives to color therapy. They wanted their work to go on and were offering what they knew to anyone who would keep the techniques alive. I agreed to incorporate their work with my own and to share it. To my regret I have never met them. Yona brought me the materials. I had a lamp made and began experimenting. Everything worked well.

As I worked new ideas came to me about how to best utilize the color lamp, infused water, food, home decor, and clothing. A full yet far-from-complete summary of how to apply color therapy appears below. Keep in mind that red, orange, yellow, magenta, and pink are warm colors. As such they activate the body's glands, circulatory system, breathing, digestive, and reproductive organs. Stimulating and energizing are their functions. These warm colors alleviate depression and other non-violent emotions and invigorate the corporeal body. They are counter-indicated in fever, delirium, inflammation, diarrhea, nervous disorders, or mental chaos. If a person is confused or forgetful, do not use red light even if the illness you are about to treat calls for it. Orange is the alternative. Orange is the best choice to neutralize confused or spacey states of mind while healing conditions that are normally treated with red. In extreme stress brought on by emotions, panic attacks, and unreachable memories of trauma, orange is a better choice than red. It is a combination of two out of the three colors that make up the lifeforce.

Cooling colors, violet, green, blue, turquoise, and indigo soothe and tranquilize. Their function is astringent and sedative, bringing pain relief and restoring calm. Cooling colors are usually indicated in cases of eye, ear, nose, and throat disease, heart ailments, fever, infection, bleeding, and severe mental disturbance due to over-excitability. Except for green, which is a neutral color, *never* use the cool side of the spectrum in paralysis, constipation, tuberculosis, depression, or melancholy.

If a melancholy or depressed individual must have blue light to calm down a persistently itchy rash which is driving him crazy, use the blue for three quarters of an hour and then apply magenta or orange to uplift his mood. Counterbalancing in such cases is essential. Otherwise the person may become morose, suicidal, or require hospitalization for his mental condition.

Orange and green are universal healers. If you don't know what color to use, green is neutral and will never do harm. It is relaxing for the body and the mind. Orange stimulates healing and instills a joyous attitude. It is great for altering pessimistic turns of mind.

For rashes, use red as a counter irritant, green to sooth, blue to take redness and itching out. If a rash is not red all over, begin with green.

Abscesses	*blue*
Acne	*blue, indigo*
Actinomycosis	*blue, indigo*
AIDS	*green, orange, magenta*

Amebiosis	*blue, violet*
Anemia	*red*
Anthrax	*blue, indigo*
Apoplexy	*blue*
Appetite	
to increase	*yellow, orange*
to reduce	*violet*
Artherio-sclerosis	*blue*
Arthritis	
pain relief	*red*
to reduce calcium build-up	*yellow*
Asthma	*orange, red*
Balance body/mind	*green*
Baldness	*indigo, violet*
Bladder weakness	*violet*
Beriberi	*yellow*
Blastomycosis	*blue, indigo*
Bleeding all types	*indigo*
Blood	
clots, or diseases	*green*
poisoning	*blue*
pressure	
to lower	*green, blue*
to raise	*red*
increase white cells	*red*
Boils	*blue, green*
Bones broken	*orange while pain present, green to knit*
Bone marrow	*red*
Bright's disease	*blue, indigo*
Bronchitis	*orange, red*
Brucellosis	*blue, indigo*
Bruises	*blue*
Bubonic plague	*blue*
Burns	
to heal	*blue, turquoise, green*
to reduce swelling	*orange*
Bursitis	*blue*
pain relief from	*red*
Carbuncles	**blue**
Cancer	*green, blue, violet*

Cancerous condition	*green*
Carcinoma	*blue*
Cataracts	*blue, violet, indigo*
Cerebral diseases	*violet*
Cerebral palsy	*violet, lemon*
Chicken pox	*blue*
Cholecyntitis	*yellow, indigo*
Cholera	*orange, green*
Chronic ailments	*lemon*
Circulation increase	*red, yellow*
Colds	
head	*green*
chest	*orange*
to loosen	*lemon*
Colic	*blue*
Colitis	*yellow*
Colon problems	*orange*
Concussion	*violet*
Constipation	*yellow, orange*
Convulsions	*orange*
Cough	
wet	*orange*
dry	*indigo*
Cradle cap	*indigo, violet*
Cramps all kinds	*orange*
Croup	*green*
Cystic fibrosis	*orange, indigo*
Cystitis	*blue*
Cysts	*green*
Dandruff	***violet***
Deafness	*indigo, yellow*
Delirium	*indigo*
Depression	*orange, red, yellow, pink*
Dermatitis	*blue, indigo, turquoise*
Diabetes	*yellow*
Diarrhea	*violet, blue*
Digestion	
upset	*orange, yellow*
impaired	*indigo*
chronic heartburn	*yellow*
malabsorption	*yellow*

Diphtheria	*blue, indigo*
Dizziness	*green, turquoise*
Dysentery	*green, blue, violet*
Ear trouble	
deafness	*yellow*
disease	*indigo*
infection	*blue*
ringing in	*green*
stimulate	*yellow*
Eczema	*blue, green, violet*
Edema	*blue*
Emotions	
control violence	*indigo, violet*
depression	*red, orange, magenta*
disturbance	*pink, violet, magenta*
insanity	*violet, magenta*
irritation	*indigo, violet, blue*
jealousy	*magenta*
Energy	
builders	*red, orange*
relaxants	*green, blue*
Epilepsy	*orange, violet*
Exhaustion	
nervous	*yellow*
physical	*red, orange*
mental	*green, turquoise*
Facial paralysis	*indigo*
Fear	*blue, orange*
Fever	*blue, green*
Fibrositis	*red, orange*
Frustration	*green*
Gall bladder	
malfunction	*yellow, orange*
stones	*orange*
Gas	*orange*
Gastritis	*yellow*
Glandular disorders	
overactive	*green*
sluggish	*orange*
Glaucoma	*blue, indigo*
Gonorrhea	*blue, green, violet*

Gout	*orange*
Hay fever	***green, blue, magenta***
Headache	*green, blue, turquoise*
Healing	*green, orange, blue*
Heart	
arrhythmia	*green*
attacks	*green (as a preventative and in recovery)*
emotional	*magenta*
rapid	*green*
slow	*red, yellow*
valves	*green, orange*
Hemophilia	*indigo*
Hemorrhage	*indigo*
Hemorrhoids	*indigo, blue*
Hepatitis	*yellow*
Hiccups	*orange*
Hodgkin's disease	*green, indigo*
Hookworm	*blue*
Hypertension	*indigo*
Hypochondria	*indigo, green*
Hysteria	*blue*
Ichthyosis	***blue, green, turquoise***
Impetigo	*blue, turquoise, indigo*
Impotency	*red*
Infection	*blue, green, indigo*
Influenza	*green*
Insomnia	*blue, green, violet, indigo*
Intestines	
large (colon)	*orange*
small	*yellow*
Itching	*turquoise, blue*
Jaundice	***green, blue, violet***
Keloids	***blue, turquoise indigo***
Kidneys	
infection	*green, blue*
overactive	*green*
sluggish	*orange, red*
Laryngitis	***blue, green***
Laziness	*red*
Liver ailments	*orange, yellow*

Lower back pain	*blue, orange*
Lung	
bleeding	*indigo*
blockages	*orange*
fungus	*blue, violet*
hyperventilation	*indigo followed by orange*
Malaria	*green*
Mastoiditis	*blue, indigo*
Measles	*blue*
Melancholia	*red, orange*
Meniere's disease	*indigo, green*
Meningitis	*violet*
Menstrual cramps	*orange*
Mental	
agitation	*orange*
confusion	*lemon*
generic	*green*
grief	*orange*
guilt	*green*
loss of control	*yellow*
torment	*magenta*
self-confidence	*orange*
upset	*violet, indigo, magenta*
Migraines	*blue, green, magenta*
Mononucleosis	*yellow, orange*
Muscles	
to build	*green*
to relax	*indigo*
reduce tension	*green, turquoise*
strains	*green, orange*
Myocarditis	*green*
Nausea	*blue*
Nephritis	*blue*
Nerve degeneration	*violet, yellow*
Nervous	*green, magenta, violet*
anxiety	*magenta*
tension	*orange*
Neuralgia	*green, violet*
Neurosis	*violet, green*
Nose problems	*indigo, blue*
Obesity	***magenta***

Otomycosis	*purple*
Ornithosis	*blue, indigo*
Osteomyelitis	*blue*
Ovarian cyst	*green, blue*
Overeating	*green*
Pain	**blue**
in joints	*red*
Palpitation	*blue*
Palsy	*indigo*
Pancreas disorders	*yellow*
Paralysis	*yellow, red*
Parasites	*indigo*
Parkinson's disease	*orange, violet*
Pellegra	*yellow*
Phlebitis	*blue*
Phlebothrombosis	*green*
Pinworms	*blue, turquoise*
Pituitary gland	
to calm	*indigo, green*
to stimulate	*orange*
Pleurisy	*indigo, orange*
PMS	*green, magenta*
Pneumonia	*indigo*
Poison Ivy or Oak	*blue*
Possession	*indigo magenta*
Prickly heat	*blue, turquoise*
Psoriasis	*magenta, violet*
Ptomaine poisoning	*blue*
Rabies	**blue**
Rashes	*blue*
Rejuvenation	*green, pink*
Relaxation	*green, blue*
Retardation	*lemon*
Rheumatism	*blue, violet, orange*
Rickets	*orange*
Ringworm	*indigo*
Scabies	***indigo, violet***
Scalds	*blue, green*
Scarlet Fever	*blue*
Schizophrenia	*violet, magenta*
Sciatica	*blue, violet*

Sebaceous cysts	*turquoise, blue, green*
Self-confidence (low)	*orange*
Sexual problems	
lack of desire	*red*
non-stop hots	*purple*
post orgasmic shame	*green*
rape victim	*magenta*
Shingles	*blue*
Shock	*blue, green*
Sinus	*orange*
Slow learner	*yellow*
Spleen diorders	*orange, or bright yellow*
Sprains	*blue*
Stress	
mental	*turquoise, indigo, magenta*
physical	*blue*
Tachycardia	***blue, indigo, green***
Tapeworms	*yellow*
Teething pain	*blue*
Thirst (excessive)	*blue*
Throat infection	*blue, indigo*
Thrombophlebitis	*green*
Thymus activator	*lemon, orange*
Thyroid	
overactive	*indigo, blue*
underactive	*orange, yellow*
Ticks	*blue*
Tissue rebuilder	*green*
Tonsillitis	*bluc, indigo*
Toothache	*blue, or red, to counter irritate, followed by green*
Trichimonous	*blue, or green*
Tuberculosis	*orange*
Tumors	*green, violet*
Tularimia	*blue, indigo*
Typhoid fever	*blue*
Ulcers	***green, violet***
Undescended testicles	*red*
Veins	
varicose	*green*
weak	*orange*

Vertigo	*red, yellow*
Violent outbursts	*green, magenta*
Vitality lack of	*orange, red, pink*
Vomiting	*blue*
Warts	*indigo*
Whiplash	*green, orange*
Whooping cough	*green*
Worry	*red*
Wounds	*blue*

Missing elements manifest as disease or energy leakages. A person who is ungrounded and out of balance is lacking in the earth element. Someone suffering from bodily stiffness may have dammed up the flow of water in their system. An individual who seems unambitious may be operating with little fire in their energy field. If someone is missing an element in their energy field or is low in a specific element the colors you use to jump-start the spiritual, mental, or physical body are:

Fire = *true orange*
Earth = *yellow*
Water = *milky white*
Air   = *pale green, or light blue*
Ether = *golden*

Silly people or those viewed as flakey may have insufficient amounts of the air element or the earth element so you will have to try more than one to see if your appraisal is correct. Begin with yellow light and observe whether or not that rebalances them. If it fails to work after five consecutive treatments change to pale green. If you are using a color lamp, one hour a day is sufficient to affect the person you are treating.

9
CRYSTALS

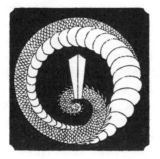

Crystals

Ancient civilizations on our own continent held crystals in such great respect that only the initiated carried and used them. Everywhere on earth in caves and on mountains there are crystals of varying mineral formations. Quartz, the most familiar, is six-sided and varies from clear to milky, purple to smoky and dark yellow. Other natural crystalline healing minerals are emeralds, tourmalines, fluorites, sapphires, topaz, aquamarines, Herkimer diamonds, and rubies. The famed Celtic healers sent to Switzerland for Morian, a dark brown smoky quartz crystal, although the smoky quartz mined in the Cairngorm Mountains is as superb for healing. The Tibetans esteemed the sky-blue turquoise from Persia over their own blue-green variety. Modern day healers show off their Brazilian quartz, claiming it purer and better than the excellent Arkansas crystals used for centuries by Native American medicine people. What is not local is esteemed.

Until the mid-nineteenth century, gemstones were believed to exert a great influence over mankind. Legends were built connecting them to astrology, healing, magic, and spiritual practices. Kings, popes, and other religious leaders wore rubies, sapphires, and emeralds in their crowns to enhance their personal power and magnetism;

although the stones were often polished into facetless cabochons, they still emanated the properties associated with them.

To the medicine people, seers, and shamans went the task of correctly mixing the right stones to give the wearer optimum charismatic charm. Each one was assigned to a specific day of the week or a planet in the heavens, and particular endowments were linked to every variety of crystal and stone. Amazingly, there is great agreement from civilization to civilization as to the special properties inherent in each type of jewel. However, debates continue to this day on the astrological association each stone carries. The healing energies and the powerful charm each stone brings with it are more easily demonstrated or refuted by the individuals who practice healing and utilize the gem's influences for personal or community gain.

Naturally, faceted stones are often prized for the shape, color, and clarity they bear straight from the earth. With higher interest in even semi-precious stones, more cutting and shaping is being done by middlemen before the gems come to market. Broken crystals are cut and reshaped with perfect points; ordinary ones are double-terminated (pointed on each end), hexagonal ones are cut square along the body with double pyramids at each end. All the tinkerers with nature claim that their work improves the ability of the stone to heal. It does skyrocket the price. But a good quality stone that you like will work just as well without adverse affects on your budget. While crystal healing usually refers to members of the quartz family, any one of the stones named here can serve in a healing capacity. All are crystalline formations though widely varying in shape, coloration and mineral content. Some naturally faceted stones employed for their fine healing, protective, and attracting qualities, are listed in the table below.

Naturally Faceted Stones

Type	Color	Function
Aquamarine	*aqua* – helps with spiritual attributes and practices	
Diamond	*black, blue, yellow, pink, clear, blue-green* – all offer protection	
Emerald	*green* – heals the eyes, cures many diseases	
Fluorite	*purple, yellow, white, clear, aqua* – wards off radiation; place between yourself and your TV or computer	

Type	Color	Function
Garnet	*red, green, pink, reddish brown, reddish purple, black, orange, dark yellow* – protection, balances second chakra and sexual organs, forewarns of danger to wearer, averts violence	
Herkimer diamond	*clear or clear with inclusions of black or yellow phantoms* – induces prophetic dreams and ones that increase self-awareness.	
Quartz	*clear, yellow (citrine), purple (amethyst), whiskey (cairngorm), black (Morian), smoky, rose (pointed hexagon is exceedingly rare)* – heal various aspects of body/mind spirit; citrine assists meditation	
Ruby	*red, green* – balances sexual energies and self-worth: second chakra	
Sapphire	*blue* – heals the mind and spirit, aids intuition: sixth chakra stone.	
Topaz	*yellow, blue, golden orange, red, white, pink* – balances neurological system, increases energy, reduces stress, harmonizes third chakra	
Tourmaline	*pink, green, pink and green (watermelon), blue, pink and blue, brown, magenta, honey-yellow, lemon-lime, red, black (Schorl)* – with the exception of black, which protects the wearer from negative interchanges, all the Tourmalines work on various aspects of the heart chakra.	
Zircon	*water clear, reddish-brown, green, yellow, blue (only when heat treated)* – the reddish-brown heals the liver, the others aid intuition	

Properties

Crystals grow in a multitude of formations. Each category of stone will consistently take shapes characteristic of its genus. Quartz is always hexagonal although the length, width, size, type of point, internal coloration, interior phantoms, and inclusions change from piece to piece and by geological location. Zircons have two axes of equal length and a third that is unequal. All facets are set at right angles to each other. Tourmalines are three to nine sided needles growing together like a stalk; the point is triangular. Topaz is rhombic in formation. Fluorite has two characteristic shapes, the more dramatic one being a double pyramid with two flat ends of different sizes, each one forming a base the crystal can stand on.

Crystals are the crossover point between two of the major forces in healing: light and sound. Every crystal contains its own song or note inside as well as a specialized rate of emitting and reflecting light. Crystals do not necessarily bestow goodness and all forms of healing virtues; they must resonate precisely with our own vibrational quality in order to produce the correct healing or energizing force. The sound contained by each crystal is part of the vibrational field which either appeals to the wearer or falls flat. Many times a person who has inherited stones feels better once they've been reset, only to let the gem in its new setting lie dormant and unused in a vault. This happens when the stone isn't one the new owner needs for their development or if they've failed to place the gem in sunlight to clear the less desirable vibrations of the previous wearer.

Selecting A Crystal

Individual stones contain their own vibrational rate within the frequency range of the mineral class to which they belong. Often these sounds are of a very high pitch above those our ears can hear. They can also be a chord within our hearing or a single note played at divergent octaves. The notes a single stone makes either matches our correct harmonic rate or it is of little value to us. One person may see a stone and really want it, yet another picks it up without any emotional involvement. Distinctive stones may resonate a sound that an entire culture or nation is attuned to and therefore be much coveted. People who are outsiders in that country will see the stone and feel nothing. Others may only want it because the majority desire it and use it only to belong and to own that which is envied. Still they won't be happy with that type of stone, because it can do nothing for them, to inspire or rejuvenate their life.

When picking a crystal for personal use or as a healing implement it is very important that it correctly match your own energy field.

An acquaintance, a traveling crystal dealer, lives in a step-van surrounded by thousands of crystals which he keeps divided by size and color, chemical compound and geological origin. In that van it feels quite peaceful. In spite of the calm atmosphere, it is difficult not to become excited about the prospect of touching and viewing so many crystals. On this visit I was looking for a relatively large crystal weighing more than a kilo (2.2 pounds) for my healing room. I wanted one that would purify the multitude of negative energies discharged during healings and counseling sessions. There were about two dozen clear quartz crystals of the correct size. I eliminated all the ones which did not appeal to me. I am rather fond of shovel-faced formations, those having one short facet and one long flat one on opposite sides. I also like the ones that come to an equal point. This occurs when all the faces are approximately the same length. Eventually, only three crystals were left for me to choose from. Holding a beautiful crystal with rainbows of light glimmering inside it delighted my eyes only; my hands and heart told me that this crystal was too cool and vibrationally silent for me. It didn't heat up rapidly enough in my hands. The next one felt as if it couldn't be its whole self with me. Putting it aside, I held another one, which warmed quickly. Lovely phantoms appeared inside, each facet seemed to tell a story. I felt quite drawn to this crystal and decided to take it immediately, rather than wait for one with rainbow colors. Although I was disappointed that the crystal which most easily matched my vibrational field did not have rainbows glowing, the one I purchased has withstood the test of time as a powerful cleansing and peacemaking friend.

It is a difficult task to pick out a crystal for another person unless you can enter into the vibrational force they carry. A stone that is beautiful may not have any connection with the recipient. It is not good enough that you yourself like the crystal and admire its warmth and beauty. If all you are able to focus on is a plain quartz crystal, then your prospects are limited for finding the right crystal for the situation and the person whom you wish to provide healing and comfort. Notice the area of their need: do they watch too much television or work with a video display terminal? Then a fluorite weighing 200 grams should be placed between them and the machine. A smaller one can also be hung around their neck while working. Does the individual have trouble opening their heart to others or suffer from being much too open? Then a tourmaline is the best gift. Tourmaline is the stone for our age, as it is a caretaker for the heart chakra, protecting and balancing it.

If people have sexual problems or have been the target of violence, a garnet can offer protection. Amethyst is the stone for a person requiring help in screening out psychic attacks. Citrine helps with meditation, hooking up the mental and spiritual aspects of your being. Clear quartz, correctly chosen, resonates with the wearer, healing all levels of their life from the physical to the astral. For broken bones, a smoky quartz strapped to the cast assists rapid recovery. The same stone ameliorates chronic health problems. Kept under the pillow at night, it works out the mental conditions supporting damage and disease.

Sapphires heal the mind and spirit by restoring your sense of proportion. Ruby is a good stone for someone with a blood disorder. Its mental and emotional qualities make you more courageous and help you to use your own power more effectively.

People drawn to aquamarines are often seekers of universal truths, interested in the mystical aspects of life. If you aren't involved in these things, then it is only a pretty colored stone. Even if you resist learning what an aquamarine has to offer, it will draw those things to you, and should you continue to wear it you will constantly experience spiritual and mystical events, which open you to the hidden realms. Eventually, your higher self will let you in on the secret of the gem and you'll either quit wearing it or become a seeker of spiritual truth.

A Herkimer diamond can be placed beneath the pillow to help you remember your dreams and also to inspire your night time forays into other realms. Other crystal formations can be used equally well to heal the mental/emotional/physical/spiritual imbalances. Emeralds are known to aid with eyesight and can heal the eyes when inserted below your pillow nightly. Worn as a necklace they facilitate tissue repair throughout the body.

Topaz is a wonderful centering device. I gave one to a girl who needed it so badly that she chipped it. Stones will absorb negative energy for you and take an injury or illness that might have happened to you into themselves. Topaz is also a great help to insomniacs, granting sleep and restfulness. It is also used for sinus and bronchial ailments.

Crystals and other gemstones run through my hands constantly. They are given to me as gifts, and when a client or friend appears to have a need for a specific one, I pass it along.

Protecting Your Crystals

Crystals do chip. It is a good practice to have a thick leather bag to carry them in. Each crystal requires its own. If they knock against one another, they will suffer breakage and/or loss of small particles. Occasionally a well-used stone will begin to have fissures near the point. This is due to all the energy it is absorbing from people during healings or in preventing injuries to its owner. To preserve your stones, either blow them clean following a healing or periodically place them in salted water for twenty-four hours. Sunlight is another time honored method of revitalizing crystals. Just set them upon a sunny window sill for a couple of days or regularly place them there following a healing. Several people claim good results from placing them in the full moon's light. Moonlight, my mentor taught me, takes away illness.

Singing Crystals

The Christmas my younger daughter was ten, she bought me a hand-sized, milky, double-terminated crystal with one water clear spot on its well shaped upper point. The lower point was partially broken. She paid one dollar for it. I kept it mainly as a gift from her, on my dresser in the sunlight for a few years. I thought a damaged crystal wouldn't do for a healing. From time to time I would clean it with my breath by blowing on the whole crystal, point towards my mouth. One bone chilling winters' day, feeling inspired, I picked it up. Holding it between my thumb and forefinger before the window, I blew on each facet while turning it counter clockwise with the other hand, six sides and repeat, six sides and repeat. After half a dozen full turns, the clear part had expanded through the crystal's entire head. Milky vapor rose up the sides, revealing rainbows of light below. More of these cleanings followed, until the the milky stronghold was in the chipped termination only. Ever after, people have told me what a fine quality crystal it is. This same crystal has served me in many capacities as a teacher and demonstrator for how crystal power operates. Although I now revere this crystal, I did not always, at least until the event recalled here occurred.

I was sharing a booth with several other healers at an annual festival where every type of electronic device is banned. Portable radios, battery operated gear and other items are always confiscated, to maintain the pre-industrial atmosphere. A client who routinely used a staff to assist him in walking missed his regular appointment, and instead met me at The Oregon Country Fair. The healing was long. At a critical moment I was drawn to use the now cleared crystal, which I'd brought along as part of an educational display of healing items. Holding the crystal over a series of muscles, paralyzed by disease, in the man's upper leg, it started to vibrate so heavily that my hand began pulsating vigorously behind it and I couldn't even hold my arm still. As I continued to move the crystal over the area, it became burning hot in my hand, the vibration becoming ever stronger. Unexpectedly, I heard a high-pitched sound resembling a piece of electronic equipment. I knew it was the crystal. I looked all around, fully aware there weren't any kids or pranksters in the vicinity. I realized the crystal could shatter; I'd been told stories by other healers whose crystals were lost in that way. Hoping to prevent this, I turned the crystal up towards the sky. Its frequency intensified. An incredible ear piercing note sounded, echoing through my client's entire body and mine as well. He looked up, startled, and I casually remarked, although I was in a semi-shocked state from hearing the crystal singing its song, "I think the crystal is working." Later he told me that when the sounds were audible, he felt sensation in his thigh's long muscles, which had been numb and unusable for thirty years.

A crystal shatters once it has given its life force to a person, destroying itself in the process. It doesn't happen often. It's never happened to me. People have told me of finding an untouched crystal reduced to powder and fragments in its usual location. Healers have also reported the destruction of a crystal during a strenuous and successful healing. And, although I've worked with crystals for years, I haven't any idea what pushes them beyond the breaking point.

To hear a crystal, place it next to your ear for a few moments. You may hear a soft melodic note or two. Do this periodically until you have heard the quartz crystal sing its song. If you own the crystal, place it next to your bed, either level with or above your head for a few nights, and ask it to reveal its sound in your dreams.

Oralee Stiles is a dear friend of mine. One year while in Portland for a book signing at the shop she and her sister Marzenda McComb own, she showed me a group of crystals found loose in a Brazilian mine. She was intrigued with the information people received from the crystals. Handing me a relatively large one to hold, she went on talking about her latest research project involving these stones. I stood in the back room, listening to a Pomo song for warriors going off to battle that I hadn't heard in fifteen years. Casually, Oralee asked if I felt anything from that crystal, because a very fine channel had said the one in my hand sang songs. Immediately, I subscribed to Oralee's Starseed Crystal Caretaker program, taking that crystal with me. It has delivered Healing Songs and Lifesongs to many students who've had trouble finding their songs in the usual manner.

The majority of the crystals have nothing to do with musical assistance. Most open the intuition of the seeker to specific information. Some do not work except for special individuals. Most are misty in color, many have inclusions or phantoms inside.*

Author Joy Gardner of Nelson, British Columbia, with whom I maintain a lively correspondence, gets together with me approximately once a year to trade discoveries. She is the author of *Healing Yourself During Pregnancy*, and *Healing Yourself*, the little yellow book found in more than 100,000 households as a handy reference. Her latest book is *A Difficult Decision: A Compassionate Book About Abortion*. All were republished by Crossing Press in 1986.

Joy had been exploring past lives with fervor and incidentally rediscovering secret practices by that means. She specifically asked to be taken to Atlantis in order to learn more about crystals. In a past life trance she saw herself entering the body of a young woman, the youngest member of a spiritual community, whose job it was to enter crystal caves, sit by a crystal until it revealed its song to her. She would then sing it's song and the crystal would come off the wall, giving itself to her undamaged. If a crystal wanted to continue to grow or remain where it was, it could withhold its song.

Contrast this with the current practice of indiscriminately bull-dozing crystals off the walls and floors of caves and hammering them apart. They become milky and sustain internal injuries from the greedy, disrespectful way they're mined.

Joy Gardner stated that,"The Atlantians were using the crystals like radio transmitters, to help spread their ideas. The old women would take the crystals to the marketplace, where they were sold as good-luck charms—much as we used to use rabbit feet. But, this was just a cover-up, an excuse to get people to take them and keep them close, where the crystals could influence the thoughts and vibrations of those who held them."

---

*For further information on the Starseed Crystal Caretaker program, write to Stiles for Relaxation, 4505 NE Tillamook, Portland, Oregon 97213.

There are ways to separate crystals by just holding them in your hands and projecting your desire. These are best demonstrated by someone who knows how to merge their consciousness with the cluster of stones. However, if you are willing to concentrate and practice on your own, you might be successful. Use no physical pressure. Stroke the stones gently as if you were petting them, while enclosing only the ones you want in your hands.

Some Idiosyncrasies About Crystals

Crystals disappear. A young mother in one of my classes related this experience with a crystal she'd lost. "An elderly woman gave me an old pendant with a large blue-purple stone in it that her father had given her. 'You'll appreciate something of this nature that you can pass on to your children,' she informed me. At the time I didn't have any children. I was living in Crescent City, California. I went away for the weekend, and where I thought I'd put this stone for safekeeping, it was gone. Just before I left I'd taken it to a gemologist and he said it wasn't an amethyst, 'I've never before seen a purple topaz but this is what it is from the weight of it.' Topaz is my birthstone. I'm used to the yellow-orange kind," the class member continued. "A neighbor's child had been over feeding the cats and I had to assume she'd taken it. I searched everywhere. I felt heartsick at its loss. Later on I moved up to Portland, with the help of a friend who had packed the contents of the bedroom. I opened up a box I knew it wasn't in because I'd been through it before, and there it was. It was only after I gave it up for lost and accepted it that there it was."

Many clients and friends have spoken similarly about losing a crystal and finding it in a location it's never been in, such as a brand-new car or a purse they'd not worn in years.

I've been able to rematerialize crystals because I wanted them back so badly. And you can probably do the same with a bit of practice. Traveling and teaching have been my lot for quite some time. Subsequent to a Sound Medicine Workshop in Vancouver, British Columbia, the woman I was staying with requested a healing. She had tumors in both breasts and feared they might be cancerous. Strictly adhering to my policy of never naming a malady, I sideskirted that issue and said she'd be all right irrespective of what the lumps actually were. As soon as the healing began, the growths seemed to melt under the small, slender, water-clear, perfect quartz I am especially fond of. After fifteen minutes it became apparent that the stone wasn't sufficient in size to totally remove the tumors in the time we had available. Setting the crystal on her shelf, I reached into my purse for the singing crystal I knew would swiftly complete the healing. It did. Short on time to reach my next destination, I hurriedly repacked my purse. Only once again at home did I find that the small crystal's sack was empty. For two weeks every time I thought of the crystal, I reconnected with it in Canada, hidden on the shelf in her room. Back less than an hour from another weekend course, frantically packing supplies for a week-long workshop while a friend's son waited to take me to the train station, I reached behind the jewelry case that serves as a storage box for remedies. There in a small velvet bag never used for that purpose, was the crystal.

Crystals will leave you if they do not belong with you. The Tule Indians say that if you lose a crystal, do not go hunting for it. If it's yours, it'll come back to you. If not, it belongs to the finder and you mustn't ask for its return. They will literally jump out of your hand if they aren't meant for the healing you are about to do. And they'll fall from your pocket or hand at other times if they're meant for another person.

Healing With Crystals

One cannot learn to heal with crystals by reading alone or by taking classes. Actually, the more courses you take, the more conflicting information you will gather. Knowing crystals is a hands-on experience. You learn by doing. Every healing opens you to more possibilities. Often, once you are working with them, dreams, meditations, and sudden intuitive flashes bring you new ideas and insights.

Quartz crystals are mainly composed of silicon dioxide—the same chemical that human beings are made of. This is a match-up in terms of energetic similarity, which might account for why every type of quartz is employed worldwide in healing people.

A Zen teacher in London had a friend with a particularly vexing problem. Jana had been seduced by her therapist, a world-renowned man who'd promised to marry her. At this point their child was eighteen months old and she was still single. As a foreign national she had immigration difficulties in Great Britain. Though she could have reported her live-in lover and former therapist to the appropriate professional bodies, she refused, always saying, "The Universe will take care of it."

To this the Zen teacher stated, "She doesn't realize she's part of the Universe."

When the situation is yours, you are the one who has to deal with it or it's very unlikely to be taken care of.

Jana purchased a large Arkansas clear quartz crystal which she placed on the nightstand by her bed. The crystal acted as a receptacle for the emotional grip the relationship had over her. At night her thoughts were cleared, and the hold her lover had on her was broken. Within a few weeks she threatened him with public exposure and he married her long enough to legitimize their child and grant her permanent resident status in England. He also provided the financial support he been reneging on during the time she'd been unable to take action.

If you don't get into your own shadow side, you won't be able to get into your saint either. Jana needed to let her power out, but she'd been afraid to see her own shadow.

An outgoing woman I'd met in the peace movement called me one evening with a horrible problem. Due to a heavy menstrual flow, prolonged by days beyond normal and debilitating cramps, she'd sought the advice of a prominent gynecologist whose only choice of cures was a hysterectomy. The woman, a former alcoholic who'd never been able to shake her addiction with traditional allopathic medicine, found success in Alcoholics Anonymous. Bravely she decided to attempt another method to cure herself of her latest ailment. She was leaving for an extended family vacation and we had little time to work together. First, I did a healing using a variety of techniques. Devising some forms of self-help for her to use on her journey was imperative. Inserting a crystal in her vagina for one hour per day offered two sound methods at the same time: quiet and rest, as well as the vibrational healing from the crystal. "A crystal used as described must not be larger than a tampon you are comfortable wearing," I explained to her. "It should have no sharp edges on the unpointed end. The point is worn up towards the cervix." Many stones can be purchased with rounded ends, or you may use a well oiled knife sharpener to patiently polish the shattered part. She shopped carefully for one that appealed to her and met the requirements.

The woman not only faithfully followed this regime on her vacation, but she also instituted some affirmations of her own choosing. Seven weeks later she returned to my office. Her most recent menstrual cycle had been comparatively easy for her (it usually worsened with travel), and her periods were getting shorter. She continued to use the crystal. She removed dairy products from her diet, since they are a major cause of menstrual irregularities. Three months after our initial visit she saw her doctor, who refused to believe her cure was anything more than a spontaneous remission. Undaunted, she wrote an article for a women's publication to let women know there are many ways to care for yourself aside from discarding your uterus.

How To Hold A Crystal When Healing

When you are healing another, grasp the crystal firmly in your hand with one of the faces completely open towards the person. The crystal will become hot in your hand once it begins working. Depending upon how well you focus energy and the rapport you have with the crystal, the heat can be immediate or build very slowly. As it becomes hot you may feel the sensation of pins and needles in your hand. And, the feeling may travel up your arm. This is nothing to become alarmed about. Should the stone begin to vibrate as well, it is a sign that the healing is progressing rapidly. The person you are working with is receiving the light and sound emanating from the crystal. A vibrating stone will move ever more quickly as the healing continues. It may shake violently in your hand; you must then hold it very firmly. Once the major portion of the healing is completed, the crystal will gyrate at a slower rate until it stops altogether. This phase is gradual and after the movement has ceased, hold it a while longer in front of the person. Tuning into their response, you will know when the healing is finished.

Every time you heal with a crystal, it won't vibrate wildly. Often it will not move at all. The feeling of heat or a flow of energy, however, is usual during a healing.

If you have a small amethyst quartz crystal with which you intend to remove a bruise or a surface blood clot (only the amethyst will dissolve blood clots), hold it so that your thumb, forefinger, and middle finger cradle it, allowing light to pour through the facets. Whether you have a small or large stone, the pointed end ought to be upright. It is desirable to have a crystal that isn't oversized for your hand. A crystal that will work well for you, regardless of the type you choose, fits in your hand as if it were molded especially for it. If you have several gemstones that work well in different situations, each one will feel exactly right whether it feels light in your hand or lies heavily. Healing with a crystal is work and you may experience tiredness and spurts of activity. Every healing is a fresh experience. Some leave you elevated and others seem routine.

Move the crystal slowly over the afflicted area. If you are not certain what area of the body is involved or you if feel the trouble is in their mind, you have two options. The crystal can be held over one temple, while the person sits upright, and you can place your other hand a few inches from the other side of their head, your open palm towards the temple. Your hand with the crystal focuses energy and the opposing hand aids absorption of the healing by keeping the energy inside the person's force field. The second way you may work is over the heart chakra with your hands facing each other on opposite sides of the body. You may place the crystal either at their back between the shoulder blades or in the front, midway above the breastbone. Your free hand is used to balance the incoming vibrations the stone and your healing hand are sending.

Whichever mode you operate in, the crystal is not to touch the person physically. The crystal needs to be four to six inches (10 to 15 centimeters) from the person. This allows the work to occur in the auric field as well as the body/mind.

There are other healing situations and conditions when it is appropriate to lay crystals directly on the body. However, this would require a great deal of instruction which is well covered by other authors. Currently a multitude of books about healing with gemstones and crystals have appeared on the market. These are recommended with commentary:

The Magic of Precious Stones is a superbly readable, extremely practical book by a highly recognized Dutchwoman, Mellie Uyldert. Published in England by Turnstone Press 1981, it is as vital in the translation as in the original.

Healing With Crystals and Gemstones by Daya Sarai Chocron, carefully lists stones by their color, outlines the way each one assists our spiritual transformation, and discusses how it heals us. The publisher is Samuel Weiser, Inc. 1986.

Healing Stoned by Julia Lorrusso and Joel Glick covers all sorts of gemstones and precious metals. I've been recommending it for more than ten years. Brotherhood of Life, publisher.

Gemstones in the Geological Museum, by W. F. P. McLintock, CB, DSc., published by Her Majesty's Stationery Office London, 1983) is not about healing, but it has the most complete information concerning the composition of gemstones, how they are tested, and where they are found. Written for the layperson, it is articulate and a valuable reference for the stone collector. The exquisite full color pictures alone are worth the price of the book. It may be purchased for £1.95 from the Geological Museum, Exhibition Road, London, SW72DE, Great Britain. Shipping costs are extra and inquiry is advised prior to purchase so that you can send money for the book and its delivery at the same time.

Conclusion

Crystals have been discussed in Sound Medicine mainly because they heal using vibration and their own internal song. A single chapter about crystal healing is barely a beginning. Much of the knowledge about crystals is still being rediscovered. The growing interest in their prophetic and healing capacities is a signal that humans may yet become the glorious living beings of Light mystics always claimed we could be.

10
JOSKA SOOS:
URBAN SHAMAN

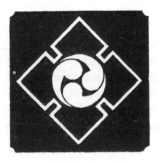

In the spring of 1985, André Christiaan Cuppen, my translator, took me to meet his teacher, Joska Soos, a shaman who works with sound. We went to a large flat in an elegant old Brussels building. In its sprawling rooms, crowded with the accoutrements of his trade, we saw Tibetan bowls, many drums, a gigantic crystal, multitudes of gemstones, a tapestry incorporating several of his artistic designs, his paintings, rattles, bells, and a dagger amongst his items. It's hard to recall everything in his dazzling display. His apartment is filled with his own paintings and drawings. Some of them have been made into large tapestries with names like, "Messager Selenite, and Ame du Papillion", (Moon Messenger, Friend of the Butterfly). He stresses the importance of art as an expression of the shamanic path.

He greeted me warmly, speaking highly about the effect the cover of my book, Companions in Spirit, had on him, since he too is fascinated by the multidimensional spiritual reservoir of the gonshe. Each of us rely on this symbol of the three in one unity concept for healing and visionary practices.

He speaks German, French, Flemish, and Hungarian. I was able to converse with his companion in Spanish. But all our interchanges had to go through André. Despite the language barrier, we were pleased to meet and felt admiration for one another. The linguistic difference kept us from having a frank discussion of areas where we disagree; I've noted a couple of those in the text.

This interview is included so you can recognize that the same components are present universally in shamanism, whether the shaman lives in an urban, rural, or wilderness environment. Obviously the tribal element is missing for most shaman, since the political climate and the onslaught of Christianity have decimated native populations. During the past five hundred years, aboriginal people have been forcibly removed from their homelands and their religions discouraged. This continues today in New Guinea, Africa, South America, and the United States. Disenfranchised by political upheaval, Joska Soos has amazingly retained his integrity and sense of proportion while becoming a globetrotting city dwelling shaman.

Joska Soos is a Hungarian shaman and artist, born in 1921. At the time shamanism, as an accepted form of healing and mystical rapport with God, was thousands of years old. It was the original form of healing, passed from shaman to apprentice, and widely practiced in the Hungarian countryside. From a local blacksmith, who was also a shaman, Joska learned to use sounds to assist people and animals in regaining their own harmony, thereby healing their physical and spiritual problems.

In his book *I Don't Heal, I Repair the Harmony* (Karnak Publishers, Amsterdam, 1985), Joska related this about his relationship with the blacksmith: "I didn't live with him, but I did spend a lot of time with him, as with a grandfather, including holidays and weekends. This was very common in a village, children were in and out of everyone's homes. I would go with him when he went to treat people and animals, to "work" on them or relieve their pain through laying on of hands or by singing. His songs didn't have words, he only sang the articulation, just the sound itself: *OEOEOEOEOEOE-OOHOOHOOHOOHRAAGH*. He believed that sound doesn't need words because the vibrations carry the meaning. He didn't go through the rational mind but made a direct connection, which isn't dependent on words, with the spiritual realm. This happens in a sort of transcendental state. It functions the same way as the beating of the heart or our breathing. It's actually a primary function which we can activate. That's not magic. Or you could say that everything is magic because it's just as much a mystery how our hearts beat or our breathing continues.

"He always stressed this and now I really understand it. One has to be open in a very special way, unconditionally receptive, not critical. Criticism must come later after enough information has been gathered. One must be able to live in a state of wonder, to be child-like. That's the necessary requirement: to be vulnerable."

During the Second World War, Joska Soos was a prisoner of war and was forced to perform hard labor in Germany. Later he went to Belgium, where he still resides. The past ten years have been devoted to shamanism and work with sound, especially the human voice. He treats people who seek him out, and teaches workshops on how people can use sound and the concepts of shamanism.

He poured me a glass of water and we both sat down at a large table in the middle of the room. His warm, healthy looking brown eyes radiated an inner glow of happiness with his life and enthusiasm for the future.

JS: Ask me anything you want, I'll answer you.

LMG: *Joska, sound is for you the most important tool in your work as a healer. Could you tell me more about sound, about the different sounds you use?*

JS: There exists an infinite number of sounds, but you could say there are three columns of sound and these are the three pillars of the entire micro- and macrocosmic types. At first I differentiate the primal sound, which can be created by using this large conch shell. It is a continuous sound that also can be made with the mouth or with a horn: *OEOEOEOEOEOE*. The second sound is a female sound*, a weaving sound: *WOEW WOEW WOEW WOEW WOEW WOEW*. The rhythm has a spontaneous effect. Then there is the masculine sound, which is a broken sound like this *BRRRRRRRRRRR BRRRRRRRRRRRRR*. Toddlers make this sound with their mouths. Why? By making this sound they create a dry, warming condition. This is a fire sound.

You can also connect these three sounds together. In all the sounds you hear, a plane, a mouse, a bird, or a human being, you can tell immediately which primary sound is involved, or what mixture it is comprised of. The uppertones (overtones) one hears so much about lately are actually part of every sound, like the primal sound. The uppertones are felt primarily in the head. They are scores of tones which sound together. Uppertones are primarily

---

*While I agree with him about the effect these sounds have, I do not assign gender to sounds.

formed with the upper palate, while the undertones are shaped in the abdomen. There are different levels where sounds are created: abdomen, stomach, chest, throat, mouth, lips, and forehead. Arabs sing primarily from the throat, nose, and forehead.

LMG: *You spoke of the masculine sound as the fire sound. Is every sound actually connected with a particular element?*

JS: Certainly! The primary sound, for example, contains all the elements: fire, air, earth, and water, plus the spirit which creates life. The undulating female sound, is a water sound. The fire sound connects with the letter R to emphasize its broken character. Various musical instruments produce the sound of a specific element. Wooden instruments are associated with the water element, whereas copper or metal instruments are indicative of the fire element. In shamanic rituals I use a rattle for the fire energy, a bell for air, and the drum for the earth. The manner one plays the instrument determines the element it expresses. For example, the element you reach depends upon how the drum is beaten. The shaman has a drum to call forth all three main sounds. Of course, the human instrument, the voice, also does this. There is a mutual influence between the voice and the element and from the element to the voice. For instance, I listen to the sound of falling water, like rain, and I connect with that sound and through it link up with the element. The shaman, as rainmaker, then sings like the rain and beats the drum, imitating thick raindrops cascading heavily plop, plop, plop.

LMG: *You also mentioned rhythm as an important factor.*

JS: Yes, sound is vibration and rhythm. Rhythm is like a container and sound is the contents. One can therefore never utter a sound without rhythm, just as one cannot talk without sound. Rhythm can exist only when sound is present.

LMG: *Could you clarify for the readers how the influence of the human voice functions?*

JS: The four elements represent four temperaments, the moods of people. Fire is the malignant temperament, air the melancholic, earth for the bloodless emotionless, and water for the phlegmatic temperaments. As you know most illnesses are psychosomatic. In healing I work with the particular temperament that is responsible for the condition, matching it with the corresponding sound element. Sound by itself is expressive. Sound has a nature. Moods are created with sound. With the right sound one can establish the psychological condition of a person.

A classic example can be found in the Bible. When David played the harp for Saul, he was trying to assess Saul's mood through the harp music. That is something shamans do. So I try to get in touch with the problems a person has by attuning to the physical, psychological, and psychic levels. A problem is a mood. I try to contact the dammed up energy, and then, using the same rhythm it has, apply sound. It's actually homeopathy through sound.

LMG: *How do you usually proceed when someone comes to you with a problem?*

JS: I have them explain what the problem appears to be. I don't invest energy in trying to guess what the problem is although I can sense the person is not balanced and whether the problem is of a physical/profane, psychological/emotional, or psychic/spiritual nature. People are relieved when they're able to communicate the underlying cause of their problem. Our modern society suffers from the fact that we can't share these concerns with each other. Or rather that we don't dare to because inferiority or superiority complexes are in the way. Many people have lost their faith in God and have no faith in human beings or politics either. That's an impossible situation. They have nothing to connect with. Oftentimes people misunderstand their problem completely. Then I tell them "Yes, that's correct from your perspective, but the situation is actually ... "

Once the problem has been stated, I begin with my shamanic transformation, assisted by instruments, including a whole series of Tibetan singing bowls. The patient sits opposite me. While drumming and making sounds, I concentrate on the main problem. Often there are side issues that will disappear once the cause has been dealt with. Using a sound range that matches the vibration of the problem creates a resonance that has the potential to restore harmony. From a shamanic perspective this technique goes back thousands of years. Yet there is no problem without a solution, no solution which doesn't create another problem.

When someone is sick in a particular organ or body part, the prototype for health and harmony still exists in the nucleus of the cells, Even when one suffers from cancer, the core of health exists undisturbed. The shaman seeks to connect with this healthy center and visualizes it as a gonshe (rotating wheel with three inner arms) of three sounds which s/he attempts to speed up to a higher frequency. Occasionally, I observe that the movement of the gonshe is very, very slow, or that it rotates in the wrong direction, or it has dropped off its axis. Then I need to correct its position and increase its speed with the aid of sound. Once I sense this, I tell the client to sing the mantra. Other sounds surface and spontaneously form a single sound, the primal sound. Then harmony is re-established.

LMG: *Is every sound a mantra?*

JS: Yes, actually everything that exists is in itself a mantra, a bundle of sounds. A real mantra is not dependent upon words. It is exclusively sound. When you laugh, that's a spontaneous mantra. We have no words to represent sighing or weeping. This is real mantra, which cannot be conveyed in words or images. Such a mantra has to occur spontaneously in whatever language you use: Hebrew, Tibetan, Hungarian, American; every language is sacred. All languages have mantras which are sung and learned by heart with the purpose of reaching a certain moment when words aren't needed anymore to express emotions, like a smile. With a mantra you liberate yourself from the representational and experience only the heart of the matter.

In shamanism you use many diverse aspects of a concept. At first, there is the word: you accentuate a word to give it a special meaning. Then you reinforce it with imagery using a sign or symbol like the pentagram or the so-called magic rune symbols or shaping motions when a priest gives a blessing or uses mudras. If this is unsatisfactory or inadequate, you move to the next step: color, just color. The symbolic meanings of color are very important since via color you reach the higher vibration of light which vibrates further into white light.

LMG: *Does this relate to sound?*

JS: When you experience sound, not through singing anymore but when you are in the sound, literally inside sound, it comes through the word, the image, colors, and light. Sound cannot be expressed without movement; the method itself is movement. The sound goes through everything but you can't start from the top. That's why, in the beginning, the word is of such great importance. Shamanism doesn't repudiate the spoken word, but you have to grow beyond the word. You have to strive to be inside the sound. This is where the true spiritualist or healer can achieve balance. His spirit is inspiring. Just his presence is enough, it's beneficial. He radiates harmony, a focused vibration to bring people into balance. When I'm in the sound, I'm apprised of the vibration of things around me whether I'm on the street or in a train. I also observe the vibration of my own spiritual problem; my incarnation is getting shorter. It's possible to fullfill my mission completely through sound. It's my spiritual goal as well as the goal of all other spiritualists to achieve the higher, finer vibrations with the aid of sound, and at the same time be of help to people.

LMG: *While working the mantra which you give to people, what is the significance of the number of sounds?*

JS: I know the symbolic meaning of numbers, but even if I didn't, it wouldn't be important. The main point is that I have found the necessary sound. You're able to enjoy a delicious meal without needing to know the caloric content. You don't even need to know how it was prepared. To achieve the sound is enough. You don't have to understand the meaning. On the other hand, we are rational beings. Westerners especially want to know first and experience later, so it's important to explain.

It's well known that when we know something and can apply the knowledge, the effect is much stronger. When a physician writes a prescription, you go to the pharmacy and buy the pills believing they'll be good for you. But had the doctor explained how the medicine worked, the effect would have been stronger. This is why in a treatment I explain the significance of the number of sounds. Seldom does the number exceed twenty-one. In most cases it's around twelve or thirteen.

The natural connection of numbers is self-explanatory. Numerology establishes something that already exists. I believe that every archetypical image has fifty complementary meanings. According to the Jewish Kabbalah, forty-nine of those are applicable to us. The Tibetans speak of sixty-four; however, they work in nuances. We don't need to go that far. We simply start with the basics. To begin, we have a mantra of seven sounds. Since the beginning of human memory and amongst aboriginals today, the number seven has been a mystic number. That's the four elements with the three polarities: positive, negative and neutral. Or it's the four character types with the complimenting polarities. Every number has its symbolic meaning and tells us something about the direction we're working with.

LMG: *Are there more ways to work with the mantras?*

JS: First of all I don't give the mantra; the people themselves give their own mantra. I observe and give them a few suggestions so they can work with the mantra. They might do a sound meditation for half an hour twice a day. They sing their same special mantra although the rhythm can be different each time. If a spontaneous change occurs in the number of sounds, you follow this alteration. While you're singing the mantra, keep in mind the problems you're dealing with. The transition from a mantra to a continuous primal sound is a physiological signal that the problem has been resolved and harmony restored.

Here are a few methods to increase your practice with the mantra. Before you fall asleep, repeat the mantra a few times. Keep it in your thoughts and sleep with it. In the morning when you rise, repeat it a couple of times mentally. It isn't necessary to chant audibly. You can chant in any circumstance that doesn't require much concentration. When washing dishes you can chant your mantra like a lullaby. On public transportation you can chant it silently in your mind. But you must remain focused on the problem or the person you're working with.

LMG: *During a shamanic ritual treatment, you have the client taste and feel the singing bowl. What's the purpose of that?*

JS: The lamas in Tibet and Mongolia do this too. The singing bowls are made of seven different metals. It's important to be acquainted with this in order to understand the effects. Symbolically, gold represents the Sun, silver the Moon, quicksilver Mercury, copper Venus, iron Mars, tin Jupiter, and lead stands for Saturn. Each of the seven types of metals has seven sounds apiece. In each singing bowl there are no less than forty-nine sounds, whether it's a large bowl or a small one. You can hear the vibration of a singing bowl even from a distance. You can taste the vibration by touching it with your tongue to experience it with your entire body. This changes your sensitivity. Later on you only have to look at a bowl to hear the sound. Evolving further allows you inside the sound when you only think of a bowl.

When I sing, I sense the presence of a large bowl. That assists me in getting into the state of sound observer. Most people become aware of their bodies only when they're sick. At a higher level, you can experience yourself as a sound being, a source of sound that is very powerful. This awareness gives me more understanding of myself, my fellow beings, the planet, and the cosmos.

LMG: *So if you experience something, you also encounter the sound of that object?*

JS: Yes, that's right. The first awareness of spirit is vibration. That's inspiration. All material things, natural phenomena or man made, everything, has the three aspects by which they are recognizable. There is the physical plane, and the caloric or radiating aspect, often called the aura. All living beings have this aspect which the rocks and metals don't have. The third aspect is the sound identity. When I am inside sound I'm cognizant of the three aspects all at once. I see a bird flying, I also see its dark blue and Bordeaux red aura and I experience its very high, shrill sound. I don't live this way, I live like everyone else in three dimensional awareness. Otherwise I couldn't stay in touch with people.

LMG: *In your book, there is a page with marks that remind me of runes.*

JS: Yes, that's the Hungarian runescript. Hungarians had their own culture when they settled there in 896 A.D. Their runes had between 32 and 36 signs. In my youth I saw shepherds use them to mark how many animals the landlords had. Even Thomas Bachi, my mentor, the village blacksmith, used a staff with runes. I'm under the impression that runes function as a memory aid. It always surprised me each time he sang differently although he always read the same thing, as if the runes served as a source of inspiration, reminding him to tune into deeper levels of awareness.

In shamanism, one works with different conscious levels. The personal awareness level goes back to conception. The genetic consciousness goes back to becoming human, and is preceded by amphibian awareness, which is seated primarily in the small brain. This in turn gives way to the water consciousness of water creatures from fish to algae to protozoa where human awareness ends. Following this, crystal consciousness begins. Air or photon awareness comes next, with energy or light awareness beyond that. The seventh level* is sound consciousness. With the assistance of runes as a memory aid, Bachi was able to concentrate on a specific consciousness level. Sound activates the connection between the seven levels of human awareness.

LMG: *Our mutual students have told me about your beliefs concerning water intake and I notice that throughout this interview you have been drinking it regularly.*

JS: People in general don't drink enough water. They need to be watchful to drink much more water in order to clear the toxic wastes in their bodies. People have problems with their intestines, liver, or kidneys due to blockages that need flushing out. It's also very important that the water temperature is as warm as the body. It is more relaxing to the internal body, soothing it through a very simple physiological mechanism. Our body temperature is 36-37 Cel-

---

*This is one of those areas of disagreement. I do not believe in transmigration and therefore have found no fish or amphibian consciousness in human beings. I assign sound to the fifth level of development reserving the seventh for Universal or Crystal consciousness.

sius (98.6 Fahrenheit) and we know that most water is at 12-14 Celsius (55-60 Fahrenheit). That's a big difference. When you drink that water it goes directly to the stomach, an important nerve center. It's where our main digestive process begins. Cold water causes contraction, cuts off the flow of enzymes, and slows down digestion. The body then has to heat that water so that it can continue functioning.

When you're tense you take a drink to create better balance. If the water is warm you're not disturbed and are better able to concentrate and remain in the moment fully. When you are occupied with spiritual matters, striving for the essence, a warmth is created inside of you. Artists in particular are aware of this. At first there is the wet warmth, you sweat. This is followed by a dry warmth and next comes a radiating warmth. This radiation is as if you're on pins and needles, which is intensely noticeable throughout the whole body. This is actually our own radioactivity. When we work spiritually, we attract more radioactivity, cosmic and earth radiation. It must be cooled off. The organism can't deal with such large doses. That's why more than a few spiritualists have died of cancer; they haven't paid attention to that fact. I'm not cognizant of drinking anymore. I simply have to otherwise I reach too high a vibration because of my concentrated work with sound. Especially the firesound, the masculine, creates large amounts of heat.

I also keep crystals in my drinking water. This practice is as old as human memory. The shamans and many religions use crystals, gems, and semi-precious stones on the body or consume them, as the Chinese did, grinding them to dust, for medicine. When you drink crystal infused water, you're drinking harmony homeopathically. Crystals stimulate our own defense mechanisms.

There is another condition that the crystal helps. The superpowers are doing underground testing. They claim the earth's crust is thick enough, and it'll easily absorb the radiation. But that is absolutely untrue. Nuclear debris radiates out, affecting the winds and other atoms which influence climate. These essential molecules are becoming very disturbed. The greatest part, about two thirds, radiates into the magna, toward earth's nucleus causing it to vibrate stronger and stronger. That pushes the radioactivity up through the earth's crust. This disturbs the climate and our very lives. When you drink crystal water, you counteract the radioactivity, consciously cooling it off. It's well known that most cancers go together with great heat in the affected organ, and that the vibration of that organ needs to be cooled down. Drinking sufficient water counteracts 70 to 80 percent of the radioactivity. With a crystal in the water there is no radiation and new energies are absorbed by the body.

LMG: *Joska, you're also a successful artist.*

JS: Yes, painting is a way to stay in touch with all levels of consciousness. Through these I live in an inspired state, which is somewhat like being in love, loving what you do. It's a perception, a true creation, something which never has existed until now. Creative people are vibrantly alive and strong, because their entire energy comes through at every level. The purpose of art is to realize the soul, that exalted vibration.

LMG: *Do you have any advice for people who want to work with sound?*

JS: Learn to listen. Listen to silence, to inner silence. When you're sitting or lying down, let yourself go, into that state between waking and sleeping. Remain conscious, not dozing. Let yourself go until your breathing and heartbeat become a distraction. Allow those sounds to go into the background, and then you arrive at a stillness, a silence, an emptiness where real things begin to happen. In the silence, the emptiness, everything has been slowed down; notice sounds, small sounds. And, of course you expand your awareness.

11
EARTH, FIRE, WIND AND WATER

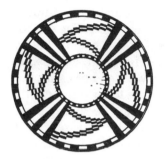

The Elements

Every one of the elements known to us has a characteristic sound. This sound carries all the wisdom contained in that element. All knowledge is accessible to us if we are willing to take the time to experience it. Reading about it cannot ever convey the depth of knowing that comes when we have rediscovered it for ourselves. This section deals with the hands-on experience of learning to control the elements. It describes many methods to hear the sounds of earth, fire, wind, and water, not only the surface sounds which we tend to ignore, but the underlying sounds. Uncovering the hidden sound within each element discloses the manner of controlling it. This is not delivered *fait accomplai* by simply doing a single meditation once in a while nor by performing it without commitment; it takes repeated effort. The sincere seeker is the one to whom knowledge falls, not the curiousity seeker. Most people require a minimum of three and a half years of devoted learning to fulfill the quest with an element.

The ability to control the elements air, fire, earth, and water is an ancient tradition in shamanism. Most shamans could master only two or three and still were considered highly evolved. The mastery of an element confers the ability to have complete control over it, not only in the world, but within our own lives. Dominance of the water element brings emotional empowerment. Wind teaches about the life force, or *prana*, confers a sense of freedom, and is the key to the mysteries. Comprehend it and you can know God's realm, hence how the Universe works. An earth apprenticeship balances the circumstances of our lives, granting everything we need to live well. Fire, in addition to burning longer with less fuel, giving information and performing trouble free, renders clear communication and power over our own thoughts. The easiest ones to learn are water and earth. Often the novice assumes knowing how the Universe works should be tackled first, but, with sad consequences, is forced to retrench and master water and/or earth. This is a warning to begin with elements that are safe to encounter and not try to outsmart the Source before you are ready. Becoming proficient with an element you also gain control over the chakra it governs. The pairings are as follows earth/root, water/sacral, fire/solar, wind/heart.

To each direction there is an element. South is the earth, west is water, east is fire and north is air. To every season belongs an element. Spring is the season for fire and air. Daily it is represented by the hours 5 a.m.-6 a.m. (5:00-6:00). Summer is the water season; its hours are 11 a.m.- noon. Autumn is a mixed season holding fire, earth, and air. The hours of the day that hold autumnal energy throughout the yearly cycle are 5 p.m.-6 p.m. (17:00-18:00). Winter controls only fire. Its hours are 11 p.m.-midnight (23:00-00:00). If you want to do the meditation of an element taught in each section and the time of year is not appropriate, you can still practice it within the hours assigned to it for each day.

Earth

There are many fine ways to unravel the intimate secrets of the earth: alternating seasons, minerals and gemstones, cave sitting, gardening, herbalism, plant lore, and specific meditations on the earth element. The lessons of the earth are visible. This element is grounding, giving you a sturdy center. It creates survival skills and removes fears about living and having. It helps your distribution of worldly goods and aids in friendships and other relationships. The study of the earth brings with it abundance, security, confidence, equilibrium, and the ability to bring your dreams and creative ideas into practice.

Methods of working with crystals for healing and knowledge were covered in Chapter 9. There are a multitide of other ways however, to master the mineral kingdom. Often plain stones, either tossed down from mountains, jagged on all sides, and smooth river-tumbled ones, yield relevant teachings to the seeker. Holding a stone while you walk can bring comfort and inner learning. The message the stone delivers may be small, but the accumulated wisdom of many stones or pebbles teaches much. If you find a rock you particularly like, take it home and keep it near you. Some people have saved pebbles and rocks since they were small children. They mayn't know it consciously, but they are learning from those rocks and transferring any undesirable mental states to them.

When I was young my Aunt Rose told and retold a family story, which was, at the time, puzzling. "My mother always said not to tell your troubles to other people. Go to the field and tell your troubles to a stone." For thirty years the advice was ignored. Living with two school-age daughters on a farm far from neighbors and friends was a trial. Heavy of heart, I crossed the meadow on my way back to the house. There at my feet was a fairly large stone. I gazed at it and lifted it from its place. Cradling it in both hands, I unloaded my entire tale. Once done I was relieved. Shall I bring it to the house?, I mused. No, that'll just bring the problems home again and with that I put it back where the earth had built up around it. My woes went away, absorbed by the stone and Mother Earth. Grandmother Laeh's wisdom, passed on to me along with her name, is now used whenever necessary.

Seasonal Changes

The cycle of the seasons is one of the keys to knowing the world. Obvious to that cycle are the changing position of the sun, moon and stars in the heavens as the planetary orbit moves around the sun. Awareness of the alteration in light from one season to another imparts a deeper perspective about the purpose of life. These things you must observe yourself over several years in order to catch the full meaning. The vibration of light reflected at the same hour throughout the different seasons contains sound. That sound is your key into the function and interaction of life on Earth. A sage may tell you exactly how it works but until you know for yourself, the words will have no meaning.

Cave Sitting

Cave sitting is not something you ought to undertake without some instruction and thorough preparation. The caves deep within the earth are a whole other dimension than the shallow sea caves found along the West Coast. People go into caves for the sound and light deprivation and the energy alteration that they provide. You can go mad in a cave or lose your way out, for once inside, your sense of direction is distorted. You cannot at times tell up from down or left from right. It is advisable not to move around too much or to go in without a flashlight and a sturdy rope tied to something secure near the entrance of the cave. There are stories in Europe of monks whose rope broke and all went deeper into the cave, believing it to be the way out, thus perishing.

There are specialized caves known to have healing properties or to invoke magical powers. One famous healing cave is the Emma Kuntz cave in Switzerland. A close friend of mine stayed within it two hours, which is considered stressfully long. He brought out fistfulls of earth with immense healing power from inside the cave. This he gave to physican friends who work with vibrational illness: sickness caused by the internal sound failing to harmonize with the person's color ray or natural sound. Sometimes it is the minerals in the cave that hold the healing properties.

Shallow caves with a back wall you can see and feel are the best for beginners. First, go to the cave during the daylight hours, taking a friend with you. Look inside and see if it is deep enough for your purposes. Any intelligent person will bring a rope, a few stakes, a long walking stick and a large flashlight. An emergency whistle around your neck and a compass are imperative pieces of rescue and safety gear. Use the flashlight to reconnoiter the walls, floor, and ceiling above you every few feet. Do not just step right into pools of water, use your walking stick to find how deep they are before you wade in. You want to obscure all light so that you aren't able to discern day from night. Go only as far as you have to in bright sunlight to be in total darkness. Getting lost isn't part of this exercise; it's plain stupidity. There will be ample opportunity to confront your fears while you're sitting inside at a secure spot for many hours. Having located a site within short range of the opening, have your friend return to the outside and have them speak in a normal voice. If you can hear it, you are likely to overhear passersby. Your friend should then stand inside the entrance and notice animals and birds nearby. If they sing or call, your friend will hear them. If they aren't audible to you, then your cave will be a good isolation zone. Your chosen cave should be in a quiet area where you won't hear traffic. Usually a cave is damp inside. It is a good idea to wrap yourself in a space blanket so that the moisture won't suck the warmth out of your body.

Assess all the possibilities. Can you drive your car and park it within an acceptable walk or hike from the cave? Do you want to be able to exit at any time? Can you find a trustworthy friend who will come call for you after a set number of days? Are you really capable of staying inside for as long a period as your ego demands you to? You aren't trying to set an endurance record. It's a learning experience for someone who is building up expertise. Start off slowly. Perhaps one day and night are sufficient. Maybe just one full day is enough. Listen to your own feelings. If you are uncertain, give yourself permission to set up a campsite near the cave should you decide that you've had it. Be there when your friend comes. Arrange a signal between you so that your friend will not go deeper and deeper into the cave in a vain and dangerous attempt to find you. As an additional precaution, make a map of the interior of the cave and give it to several people you trust, so that you are assured of being found. Most important, once you select a spot to sit in, do not change it or go deeper into the cave.

Necessities:

Several quarts (liters) of drinking water; 100 yards (92.5 meters) of rope; 50 sharp stakes; flashlight; space blanket; sleeping bag; warm clothing including a knitted cap for your head; emergency kit to be carried on your person at all times; police whistle; large size plastic garbage bag; Bic type lighter; long candle; Snickers bar to be eaten only if you are really lost or disoriented.

On the chosen date, go to the cave and set up your rope to the entry and the stakes. For safety, only go in as far as your rope stretches. Enter with your friend and recheck all the markings on the map. Sit down and be settled before your friend leaves. Turn off your flashlight. Finally you can be alone to do some intense cave sitting and begin to hear the inner sounds of the Earth. Listen carefully to the sounds inside the cave. Be still; do not sing, whistle, or otherwise make your own sounds. This is an exercise in receptivity.

If you are actually in total darkness and you see an animal clearly, then it is probably an inner animal and not a real one. Some types of cave dwelling animals emit their own light but not foxes, rabbits, or bears. Light and above ground sound deprivation will have the effect of loss of a sense of time and lead you into great intuitive information. At first you may deal with your own personality and your fears, anger at others, temporary loss of freedom, and other anxieties. The Universe in its wisdom will not deliver solutions to your personal problems that damage others or go against the higher human moral code. If you come up with a vengeful thought or action to undertake, recognize it as your own and ask for guidance and assistance to arrive at a peaceful, appropriate conclusion. Once you have successfully formed some resolve about your relative situation in life, you will be able to go on to the important insights with which cave sitting rewards the true seeker. The information and insight you receive is truly individual and will take some time to assimilate into your life. A good sitting can supply you with years of work, each piece implemented as the previous portion is successfully achieved.

Earth Meditation

This meditation is designed to let you hear the heartbeat of the Earth. After you have heard it for a sufficient amount of time, you will begin to hear it everywhere that is natural: on mountains and hillsides, in the forest, or in your own garden. Anywhere it is quiet, the inner voice of the Earth will communicate with you. The heartbeat delivers information and teaches by intuition.

Select a place where there are few people and little distraction. The quieter the site, the better for your concentration. Use different locations as you practice the Meditation of the Earth over the seasons. A mountainous area, a lakeshore, secluded meadows, open plains: each will lend another dimension to what you already know.

On a blanket made of natural fibers or directly on the ground itself, lie spread eagle, face down, one ear to the ground, arms out to the side, legs apart. You will be most relaxed this way. Breathe normally. Remain in this one pose for approximately three quarters of an hour. Then rise and sit quietly, remaining silent. Spend at least fifteen minutes in reflection. Practice this meditation as frequently as the weather permits. It will help you to tune into the inner harmony and workings of the planet we live on.

When you have mastered this meditation and can hear Mother Earth's heartbeat, you'll be able to tame an earthquake, protect yourself and others from falling rocks and shifting sands, control avalanches, direct the growth of plants, communicate with animals, and have advance warnings about earth movements and other phenomena. You will also be able to find underground caves, streams, mineral deposits, and buried objects.

Seeds And Plants

Every plant has its own characteristic sound. That is why singing over a plant will preserve it once it's harvested. You can also sing over a plant you wish to have grow stronger. Scientific research has shown that plants respond to our emotional state and to music. They also register shock when another plant is being destroyed. Communicating with plants is a simple undertaking. Anyone can energize a plant by sending it love. One of the easiest ways to master the earth energy is to have a garden and be introduced to Mother Earth's cycles, growing patterns, and wisdom through the plants you tend. This takes time, patience, and devotion. The earliest reward is fresh, healthy food and flowers from your own garden. If you grow medicinal plants, you will be contributing to your own healing powers as well.

To really know the earth through your garden, keep it organic, eschewing pesticides, herbicides, and chemical fertilizer. Get to know where the energy comes from and how the earth transforms it. If you notice a fruit tree that's ill, bury large amounts of garlic beneath its roots and watch it revitalize, gaining the ability to fight off insect invaders. When you feed a tree organically, you are improving its immune system. Composting or letting the chickens eat your household leftovers and applying their manure to the garden is a learning experience in itself. There are multitudes of excellent books on organic gardening. Let that be your winter reading to begin the study of the earth cycle early.

It may take several seasons to master the garden and learn about the earth from seeds and plants. Harvesting your own seeds for next year's crop and planting them will show you many things about genetics.

Earthy Healings

There are ancient techniques for using the earth itself in healing. At Kashia Rancheria one morning, my eight-year-old was stung by a bee. The men standing nearby said to make mud and put it over the bite. We did and it worked. Any bug bite will lose its poison to the drawing power of wet earth.

Clay is used extensively in drawing out pus, swellings, and tumors, internally as well as externally. There are many minerals in clay and each has a distinct healing attribute. The color of the clay is determined by the mineral content. The red has iron in it. Topically it removes oily skin conditions and draws deep toxins out of the tissues. Blue contains a natural calcium fluoride, which is helpful in strengthening and retoning skin. Yellow blends bentonite and iron; it aids in elimination. White is commonly used instead of talcum powder. Green clay is preferred in all forms of healing and is often taken internally. Clay you gather yourself or purchase from a non-medicinal source must be heated to 300 degrees for one hour in your oven before using it. This removes bacteria and other undesirable creatures. Michel Abehsera's *The Healing Clay* (Swan House Publishing) is an extremely well written, concise, practical guide to using clay in healing.

If you sustain an electric shock, the very best remedy is to bury the affected parts of your body in earth for half an hour. This draws out the undesirable electromagnetic field the electric current brought into your body. The electricity in the wall is very different from the type we have flowing through us.

Sand is the preferred medium for dealing with arthritis and rheumatism. Bury yourself with the help of a friend in very warm sand. Do not bury your head. Cover all areas afflicted with arthritis or other joint pain. Remain three or more hours, weather permitting. If the sand next to your body becomes damp and cold, end the treatment at once. Remember to take liquids while you're buried and afterwards. The sand may drain fluid from your body as it removes the substances causing your condition.

Water

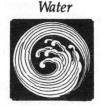

Water is the most important substance in the world. Without it we couldn't live. Anatomically, we are 90 percent liquid. Deprived of moisture, we would shrivel away. Human beings are forever taking in and eliminating liquids from their bodies. Fluids in the form of sweat, urine, and saliva are constantly excreted. Quenching thirst, breathing (20 percent of the body's aqueous intake arrives through the lungs), and washing, daily carry water to our organs and tissues. Water also washes away impurities.

Rainstorms often alter the weather, relieving heat spells. They also give the crops nourishment. Fog protects fruit trees in the cold and prevents freezing weather from entering geographical locations where it's misty blanket has spread. Water is a very changeable element. It can be as silent as snow, as loud as hailstones, as devastating as a raging river suddenly swollen, overrunning its banks, as calm as a lake without wind. It alternates from breakers far offshore to swallowing landmarks in ocean storms, and with a steady, persistent drip, drip, drip can wear away any geographic formation.

If you are a strong swimmer who takes to lakes, bays, and other natural bodies of water rather than a pool full of chlorinated water, you're intimately acquainted with the frequency of the element. Mastering water would be a natural extension of your lifestyle. Even waterskiers show an affinity for the element, but it's nearly impossible to get close to the water's sound while behind a motorized vehicle. Surfers often wind up on a spiritual path from having meditated upon the ocean while waiting for it to deliver the perfect wave.

The Meditation of Water is how we learn to control fog, rain, snow, hail, floods, clouds, drought, and our own emotions.

The Meditation Of Water

On a dry day in sunshine or clouds, go to a creek or river without much foot traffic, removed from roadways and industry. This is the best choice for water meditation. A place where the water is in obvious motion, whether it runs swiftly or bubbles slowly over the rocks—a rapids, a waterfall, however small, as long as it is one that doesn't come out of a drainage pipe—all of these are good settings where you are likely to succeed. Wherever the flow has been tampered with (e.g. a dam or aquaduct), avoid that spot, for it will not have the characteristic sound of water.

Find yourself a dry place to sit comfortably, close to the water's edge for you must look at it with half closed eyes as well as listen. Chose any seated position you consider agreeable for a prolonged period. If your site is wet, you ought to have impervious material under your blanket. Becoming chilled, even in summer, is a possibility and warming up afterwards can be difficult. In all events, take good care of your physical body, and exercise the precautions enumerated here. **Warning:** Do not under any circumstances enter the water. Doing so will spoil the meditation session and it can be dangerous as well. The water will call to you and you must resist.

Once seated in a pose, remain that way for twenty minutes, staring into the water and listening to its characteristic sound. Merge with that sound. After twenty minutes (do not bother to bring a watch, this is measured by internal time and a watch will interfere seriously with your progress), cover your face and head with a shawl or towel. Turn away from the water and rest. Ten minutes later remove the head covering. Sit in a position that is easy for you again, and repeat the exercise, steadily gazing at the water, ears attentive to its underlying sound. Stay this way for twenty minutes and then rest for ten minutes, turning away from the water and covering your head. During the pauses you will hear the water, but less intensely. The third time and last time you look at the water for twenty minutes, becoming one with the sound. End by leaving the place where you've been sitting. Go to a spot where you can lie down and cover your head so as not to be disturbed by outside noises. Don't leave for at least half an hour. In this way, the energy and sound carried in the water integrates with you. Repeat this practice as often as you wish, until you understand the basic principles of water and have mastered them.

Ocean Ritual

This is a an offering made to the ocean to have wishes granted. Go to the seashore at dusk, taking a candle, some incense, tobacco, flowers, and other offerings you feel the ocean would appreciate. If you are a smoker, refrain from smoking until you have left the beach. Forgo plastic or other substances that aren't biodegradable. You must show respect for nature if you want her to help you. Asking for the restoration of health, or the removal of bad habits, or an end to a drought or excessive rain, world peace, and other non-material needs works best.

Dig a hole on dry sand nearest to the incoming tide. Make it large enough to hold all your offerings securely, but not deep or too wide. Taking care, arrange your offerings in the hole. Light the candles and incense. Make your request. Prayers are best said from the heart even if they are simple. Those that are sincerely made on the spot are better than flowery words another has put in your mouth. Once you have said your prayers, leave and don't look back to see if the ocean has taken your offering. Should you glance again all your effort will be wasted.

If a large wave moves in and floods your offering site while you are lighting the incense or saying your prayers your appeal has been granted. Leave immediately, averting your eyes, and be grateful that your request has been so eagerly received.

Taking To The Waters

Water is famous for its healing and transformative powers. People drink mineral water from specific geographic areas for their health. Many prefer spring water, which is flowing over still water due to the energetic level the former contains, as well as the reputation spring water has for purity.

Running sweet water and the ocean contain frequencies that are superior for healing and purification. The salt content of the ocean resembles that of blood, the liquid organ of our body. The sea is well known for its curative powers. Soaking an injured or infected body part in the ocean is an age old technique. Swimming in seawater will open boils and other infections rapidly, letting them drain and heal. It also helps in recovery from severe bruises and muscle strains.

Many years ago a friend asked me to bring back a bucket of seawater for her dog, who was limping. I was going to the ocean anyway and all it required was to take along leakproof, covered containers. Her pet cooperated by sticking his leg in the briny water and standing still for half an hour at a time. He recovered within a few days from the injury he'd sustained.

The ritual healings I do are often held by a spring or freely moving creek. The vibration of the water, as well as the water itself, carries the disease away. In these healings the client rarely has more than a dab of water poured over their head to remove thought patterns that contribute to ill health.

The next method was used by Native Americans for centuries before Europeans reached North America. Let the water run into your cupped hands, filling them. Throw the water over your forehead and crown three times, allowing it to drip down your back. When you've been in an argument, had an intense day, be it good or bad, been ill or injured, when you're emotionally overwrought, this technique will alter your vibrational output, restoring calm and order to your body, mind, and spirit.

For asthmatics the water cure method is rather harsh. The river needs to be a very cold one, where the mountain snows melt into the tributaries. First their entire body is rubbed with river or creek sand. Then they jump into the icy water and stay totally submerged for about eight to ten seconds. Lifting their head above water, they remain in a couple of minutes. After that they dry off by rubbing their entire skin surface with a rough towel. If done regularly the asthmatic condition will not ever degenerate into attacks. Once a month will improve the resistance of the immune system. Cold ocean water has the same effect.

Whether you are by the seaside or a river, make certain the place you are about to use is not treacherous. The river needn't run swiftly or be deeper than knee level where the person enters. The ocean ought to be free of sleeper waves and undercurrents. Know your beach area before subjecting yourself or another to danger.

Singing by creeks will send your message down the creek and out into the world. When a person is ill or emotionally unbalanced, singing for them next to a body of running water adds to the curative powers of the song. The underlying sound of water itself is healing.

Even a weak person sitting next to a river or creek can gather strength from it. The amount of time they spend depends upon the weather and their general condition. Fifteen or twenty minutes are the limit until a person gathers strength. As they become accustomed to being by the water, the time can be extended. The faster the water runs, the more its energy output will be. A site that has slow moving water lengthens the amount of time a debilitated individual can stay there. If they are able to speak, listen to their desires. If they aren't, observe them carefully for clues of overstimulation that resembles exhaustion.

Your thoughts and prayers are strengthened by the proximity to water. Chanting or singing beside creeks or rivers can deliver you to a deep trance state wherein your clarity and perceptions are heightened. This will improve your telepathic powers not only in that moment but for the period immediately afterwards. If you keep silent about your newfound ability, it's likely to last longer between water sittings. Before acting on what you receive clairvoyantly, check it out in the real world. As any sensible person would do with a new skill, proceed cautiously. Send messages while sitting near the streaming water and see if they reach their destination.

Ocean Listening

The ocean provides a combination of wind and its own roar. On windy days, the sea is much wilder than on calm ones. To learn the sound of the ocean, go on clear days, rainy ones, at wildly windy times, and also listen to it when the soft gentle winds blow. A variety of experiences are necessary to understand the power that drives the oceans. Inside the sound of the ocean lies one of the mysteries you may uncover by persistently challenging yourself to stay on the shore while hearing the waves, whether they pound or lap the beach. Scout out different coastal formations, cliffs above the surf, sea caves, dunes, open barrier beaches, and hidden coves. The sea will sound many ways depending upon the nearby geography. Keep mindful of the tides to prevent being caught off guard by the advancing sea with no avenue of escape. In every exploration regarding the elements, exercise good judgment.

Listen to the ocean at any time of year. In the winter, when it freezes in northerly latitudes, you may observe an unusual phenomenon. The sea does not freeze over as do other open bodies of water due to its salt content. It boils and that boiling has a sound like no other.

Fire

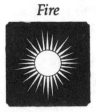

Fire is a transformative element. Fire cooks, changing the color, consistency, taste, and aroma of foods, blending all those that are put in the same pot. It frees us and enslaves us, which is a paradox. Since industrialization, fire has been very easy to come by. It's as simple as striking a match. In previous centuries, fire was faithfully guarded and attended to once begun. The firetender would carefully cover the coals with ashes so sparks burned until morning when fresh fuel rekindled a roaring blaze. If the fire went out it meant half an hour or more of work with flint and sticks to light again.

Because we have easy access to external heating methods, we no longer know how to perform *tumo*, the art of inner fire. Outside on icy days we do not know how to heat ourselves without dashing into doorways or applying layers of clothes. When stuck in traffic on account of snow or waiting for an overdue fuel delivery at home, we are just plain cold. The early civilizations in Northern Europe wore only rudimentary coverings, even in winter. American Indians did not have extensive wardrobes. They frequently wore only a warm blanket or shawl to retain body heat. Tibetan monks took initiates to freezing waters naked and wrapped them in wet cloths, which they were required to dry on their bodies. This was done repeatedly, and the faster a devotee dried his remnant the greater his proficiency at tumo became. Teenagers often display this capability, to the dismay of their elders, who believe they will catch a chill in such scant attire. Yet their inner fire is quite hot, and if left alone, they may acquire the ability to remain warm in weather that sends their parents to the furrier.

Speech is a component of fire. You might notice that during a lengthy conversation, your body temperature rises. Occasionally, you may even feel vaguely ill following intense or prolonged talking. Speaking rapidly evaporates liquids. That is one reason long talks over coffee or tea are so popular and well ritualized. Control over fire gives you control over your own words. Your communication becomes temperate and each phrase has meaning. Mastery of fire grants immunity from verbosity.

Fire is an integral part of all civilizations worship practices. Traditions of eternal lights kept aglow in churches and synagogues remain, as does the custom of lighting commemorative candles to remember a departed loved one. Candles are usually burning on the altar during services. Public bonfires were held throughout Europe on these days before the advent of Christianity subverted the old spiritual order: August first, October thirty-first, February first, May first, summer solstice, spring and fall equinox. The only exception was the Yule log, which was burned indoors for ten consecutive days between winter solstice and New Year. Most of these days are still important to us, but the fires aren't as widespread. Once a year, Switzerland still has public fires in every hamlet and city to celebrate Swiss Independence Day which coincidentally happens to be the first of August. In America, Halloween is a very big night of revels and fun, although the fires are mainly confined to the inside of a pumpkin's head.

All Night Fire Sitting

Open fires burning all night have the power to break down our resistance to change. They serve as a clearinghouse, allowing new thoughts and fresh ideas to circulate in our overly packed minds. We all hold far too much useless information in our heads, blocking intuitional and inspirational forces. A fire watched and heard in silence is one painless way to open yourself to higher thoughts.

If it is a cold or rainy night, the fire should be held indoors in a fireplace. It can be held inside a tipi if you have one available. But by no means ought you indulge in any unsafe activity, especially building a temporary shelter with unproven fireworthiness which might turn into a death trap. If you have no fireplace or tipi, wait until it's not inclement weather, and build your fire at a public campground or use your own hibachi in a secluded backyard.

You begin the fire as close to nightfall as possible, which means you'll have a longer fire in January than you will in March. Make certain you have enough fuel, either wood or coal, to take you through until daybreak. Many people can sit watching the same fire if they all maintain absolute silence, and each has an unobstructed view of the fire. This is a good group activity. Only one person acts as firetender throughout the entire night. No one else is to touch the fire under any circumstances. It is imperative that the firetender remain awake and alert at all times. If the energy of the firetender falters, then the fire will reflect this. In a ceremonial fire, there is no firescreen to protect you from sparks and falling wood. Therefore, remove rugs and other combustible items from directly around the fireplace. The firetender sits close to the fire, minding it constantly to keep it blazing brightly all night long. The only reason to move from that spot is to get more fuel. The firetender for a group can double as the one who makes certain that the others stay awake or that task may be assigned to another individual. Being the firetender is a great honor. Choose someone with enthusiasm, dedicated to achieving the goals of fire sitting.

Always build the fire in a respectful manner. The less talking the better. Begin with a square interwoven of long pieces of wood. The sticks and paper to ignite the fire are placed along the bottom rungs of your wooden weaving. You can use the native American method of keeping it going. Once the square has burned down to knee level, place long logs on top of the burning wood and hot coals. As each portion is consumed you push the remaining part further into the fire. Replenish as necessary.

Whether you have made an indoor fire or an outdoor one, seat yourselves quietly maintaining complete silence, and watch the fire as fully alert as possible. Hear the fire as it progresses from wild flames, to embers and then becomes intense again when fuel is added. This is a special meditation which will leave you with insight, emotional and mental clarity, and renew your spiritual life. You will see your emotional gamut from sadness, to fear, to anger, to shock, to mirth, to calm acceptance, surge upward from the unconscious at different moments. Let these run their course. You may have incessant mental activity for part of the night and then it will cease. From that point forward, intuition is functioning. Notice what your higher self tells you. The crackles, pops, and general sounds a fire makes as it burns serve as signals from your unconscious to your conscious self, reflecting your internal psyche. Your soul level in speaking to you may tell you to sever an association, but never to harm anyone. Everything you learn from fire sitting is to be seasoned and subsequently re-examined. One essential thing you must learn about visioning is it can take as long as ten years to actualize what you receive. But it will be done with benevolence toward everyone concerned.

A therapist I know accompanies his clients to a wooded place and has them gather the materials to make a fire. They then build the fire without any instruction from him. He watches the fire, and from the intensity, coals, coloration of the flames, the type of sparks it sends out, and the sound it makes while burning, diagnoses the analysand's internal fire and the basic course of treatment they'll require.

Some common sense tips:

Wear warm clothing. Your body temperature will drop during the night, and without extra clothes you may become chilled in spite of the fire's heat. Keep a blanket handy.

With an outdoor fire, use an impervious ground cover to keep the dampness from seeping through into your body.

Drink black tea throughout the night. Fire dries out your body fluids. The tea will also aid you with wakefulness.

Seat yourself in a comfortable manner to enable you to remain in one position for an extended period of time. It's best not to move around or fidget too much while watching a fire or doing any other spiritual quest.

Warning: Remain alert or you may be caught in one of the inferior emotional states the fire raises. Sparse periods of dozing are not uncommon. These are part and parcel of the visioning experience, but if you actually fall asleep for long stretches your quest will be aborted, and you will have to deal with many of the unresolved emotional components in the waking state for weeks to come.

Meditation Of Fire

This meditation will yield power. Once aware of fire's ways you can read messages and pictures, hear the songs it sings, and touch its life force as it breathes. Meditation on fire teaches clarity of words. Your word is your fire. The fire meditation is for controlling fire and our own thoughts. Once we control fire, our words are well selected and communication is easy. In every spiritual or religious practice fire is known as the representative of God.

The seasons of the year for this activity are winter, autumn, and early spring. The times of day to begin are 5 a.m. to 6 a.m. in the morning, 11 a.m. to noon or 11 p.m. to midnight (23:00-00:00). The entire exercise takes one and a half hours. Early in the morning or late at night are the most fruitful periods, when you are least apt to be interrupted. While the fire is in progress, do not answer your telephone or doorbell. Parents, take care to do it at a time when your children are unlikely to require your assistance.

Build a good sized, but not dangerous fire. Restoke it only once. No fire screen is to be used, for the view must be unobscured in every way. Even glass doors will intercept your meditation, unless it is a single panel without handles.

Sit at eye level with the fire, so that you may gaze fully at it. Sit either cross-legged or kneel on a cushion with your elbows on the floor and your hands supporting your face. If your physical condition precludes floor sitting, you may use a low, straight backed chair. This will keep your eye contact with the fire steady.

Stare at the fire without moving for fifteen or twenty minutes. Then turn and look away for approximately ten minutes. Refuel your fire and resume gazing unflinchingly at it for the same length of time. Then turn away and rest for about ten minutes. The third and last time, look at the fire for fifteen or twenty minutes. Remain quiet for fifteen minutes after the last round, reflecting on whatever issues the meditation has raised for you. If you have chosen to fire gaze late at night, you may go directly to bed after tamping down the fire and replacing the fire screen.

If you do this meditation daily for three months, you will attain mastery over your speech and be able to put your hand in a fire without getting burned. You will also notice a measurable increase in your mental and physical energy.

Wind

The wind is the one planetary element that has no boundaries. Every nation feels the same wind. It takes about two weeks for air circulation to go from the Tropic of Cancer to the Tropic of Capricorn. As the disaster of Chernobyl amply demonstrated, we are truly one world and whatever is released into the air travels everywhere. What is it then, that permits us to destroy the very air that we breathe? We can fast for prolonged periods without damage and, if it is done sensibly, become healthier in the process. We can go only eight days without water in a normal climate. In the desert, a shorter period would completely dehydrate the human body, destroying it. Yet air, which only the most renown mystics can suspend inhaling, is the absolutely crucial. Denied air, we would live not more than eight minutes. Surviving oxygen deprivation often entails loss of brain function and motor coordination.

Accounts of the deadly effects acid rain has upon plant life, the air pollution traffic causes in our overly populated cities, or the ever greedy corporations who misuse our shared resources as their private dumping ground, has had little effect on enforcement of public policy. Until oil, gas, and electricity replaced kerosene and coal, the most prevalent disease was tuberculosis. Modern medicine didn't cure it. Removing the chemical irritants that undermined the immune systems of weaker people ended the reign of TB. Just as this chapter emphasizes control of the elements, look at the wind and the quality of your precious breath, and take steps to insure that life on Earth will go on. Controlling our environment means making waves, persuading your fellow beings to think beyond the moment and their own immediate gratification.

Each wind is related to a season: East wind/spring, South wind/summer, West wind/autumn, and North wind/winter.

It is not recommended that you undertake the wind without first mastering earth or water, unless you are well-seasoned at sailing a wind powered vessel or an alpine mountaineer with much expertise. Prior to setting about controlling the wind, it is strongly advised that you have a spirit guide to accompany you. *Companions in Spirit* by this author will provide you with all the instruction and information required to locate your own spiritual allies. Once you know and trust your guide, you may proceed to learn about the wind from a mystical standpoint.

Wind Meditation

Locate a place where there are few trees, and none in your immediate vicinity. High on a hillside with an unobstructed view, on a flat plain, by a large lake with natural surroundings (no houses or busy parks), you will be alone and hopefully undisturbed. Wherever you choose to be, you must have complete access to the sky; you shall be staring into it throughout the meditation. Naturally, you will not look directly at the sun, since this would permanently blind you.

A warm climate is a prerequisite for the meditation. Prepare yourself by fasting for two days prior to your journey with the wind. This exercise is not for early spring or late autumn, when the weather is too unpredictable and may rapidly turn chilly. Fasting may include drinking herbal teas or unsalted vegetable bouillon. No solid food should be eaten.

On a day with relatively high temperatures, leave your home early and go to your site. Bring a blanket to sit or lie upon, a head covering, and a thermos with tea or hot water in it. Take the emergency kit spoken of earlier. Preferably the day will be a windy one, the more wild, the better to hear the sound as it blows. You may sit or lie in any comfortable position. If the weather turns cold, sit up and pull your knees to your chest. This posture preserves body heat. Once settled, listen intently to the sound of the wind and gaze at the sky. Let the sound envelop you. Phenomena may occur during the wind meditation. Beings of light may appear, unfamiliar geometric designs, patterns of the wind approaching and receding, flashes of information, and visitations from the entities who control the element. These you watch and listen to, but above all concentrate upon the underlying sound of the wind. From time to time throughout the day, cover your head, relax totally, and remove yourself from direct contact with the wind. Remain until dusk. Then go to your home or a quiet, previously rented room and be by yourself. Do not write, read, or play the radio or television. Stay with the sound of the wind so that you can absorb its power to the fullest extent.

Stargazing

Stargazing is an ancient method of divination. Shepherds in the time before written history were said to lie awake in their outdoor beds looking at the stars and receiving prophetic visions from them. The Mayans, Egyptians, Babylonians, Chaldeans, Hindus, and Chinese all practiced forms of astrology that evolved from star gazing. At the time America's indigenous peoples were conquered and subjugated by the pioneer settlers, the Navajos were still teaching their young to read the future by stargazing.

To spend a night under the stars is an endurance test. Any starry night will do. Winter or summer, spring or autumn, you only quit if it rains heavily or clouds totally obscure your view. Whatever the weather, dress appropriately and wear more warm clothing than you think you will need. In an open meadow where there are no electric lights and only the heavenly bodies shine, lie or sit looking directly into the sky. A full moon cuts down on the number of visible stars, but it too portends the future. Stay in your place without moving, watching the celestial progression overhead.

As with every practice, the more firmly you approach it, the better your results will be. The development of prophetic skills is enhanced by repetition and careful consideration of the data you accumulate.

Songs In The Wind

Day or night, you can go outdoors in sparsely populated areas, listen quietly, and hear ancient voices singing in the wind on Indian land and former Indian land. The songs are the type covered in Chapter 4. They are in languages beyond recorded time. These songs sung into the air by long gone peoples still ring out their prayers centuries later. When the wind is furious, it bellows out the songs faster. A calm wind sings the songs slower. Every area seems to have its own cadence, vocables, and music. The songs are endless. They will be sung as long the wind blows.

Chant For The Elements

The earth the fire the water the air
returns, returns, returns, returns
The earth the fire the water the air
returns, returns, returns, returns
The earth the fire the water the air
returns, returns, returns, returns
Hay ya ya ya ya ya
Hay ya ya ya ya yo
The earth the fire the water the air
returns, returns, returns, returns
The earth the fire the water the air
returns, returns, returns, returns
The earth the fire the water the air
returns, returns, returns, returns
Hay ya ya ya ya ya
Hay ya ya ya ya yo

12
THE HEALING SILENCE

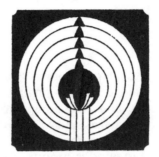

Silence

There is a natural silence so incredible that human beings are in awe of it. It is known mainly in northerly latitudes during wintertime. The very air is alive with stillness after a snowfall. Until the streets are cleared and motorized vehicles can run again, even a city is silent. Snow silences birds and other animal calls. Animals, impressed by the intense quiet, become still in order to not give away their presence. The peacefulness the snow brings is a spectacular gift.

The dead calm before a storm is another type of silence; one filled with anticipation of events to come. Whether it is a thunderstorm or a regular cloudburst, rain clears the atmosphere, leaving the world fresh. More violent storms also unleash a pristine stillness afterwards, but often the damage they've done outweighs the silence, and it isn't as appreciated.

The silence of frozen rivers beyond the city limits is another phenomenon to be enjoyed in winter. Only the crunch, crunch of your boots can be heard as you walk. If you stand still all is silent.

Early in the morning beside a calm lake in summer you can find that same special quality of silence, if the other campers are asleep or are nature enthusiasts like yourself. During sundown, just before darkness falls and the animals come out you can bask in a hush broken only by an occasional jumping fish or otter swimming.

On Sunday mornings, the financial districts of major cities are the most silent canyons. Before ten in the morning, you are so alone you might feel like the last living earthling. A late night walk through the business area after working hours produces the same stillness, broken only by your footsteps echoing through the abandoned streets.

Silence, that all too infrequent quality of modern life, is essential to our emotional, mental, physical, and spiritual growth. Without tranquillity we live in a vast network of co-conspirators sucking energy rather than giving inspiration and innovation a chance. To tune into the Universal Life Force, human beings require privacy, quiet, and the desire to listen to that small voice within. In nature, we who have grown so far away from our earthly roots in overly orderly suburbs or congested cities, glued to our work and the ubiquitous television set, can be healed and held in unconditional love.

Fear of silence, the dead places in conversation that help us to rearrange our thoughts, forces talk that has little depth. Fright of hearing what the inner voice might say, keeps people from enjoying quiet that can be enlightening. Silence in the early morning hours, before the city wakes up or the sun shoots its colors across the sky, prior to the stars falling asleep, is the best time to meditate. That is the deepest silence that can be had on Earth. It is worth rising early to hear the voice of the Creator in that stillness.

The Voice and Silence

In the early '70s, my friend Mitzi Linn lived in a remote mountain cabin in the Southern Oregon woods. In the silence her lifestyle afforded, her voice and her music channeled through her. Parking on the road below her house you would often hear her singing strongly. During that time she composed quite a bit of very fine music. She believed that music was meant to be a healing tool and personal growth experience. It was her meditation. Now she lives in the city, her profession is reader, healer, and teacher. She still sings robustly, but not as many hours a day, and she has learned to use her voice to help heal others. She alternates singing her personal healing songs to her clients, chanting, or making sounds with over tones like Siberian shamans; in truth, using whatever seems intuitively appropriate for the situation. Her classes in women's spirituality and the ancient goddesses feature these techniques as well as her own singing.

Of the benefit silence affords to bring out your inner music, Mitzi Linn says: "Everything comes out of silence. When you get silent enough and go deep enough, your voice will find the perfect note(s) or pitch for you, one(s) that express your particular vibration. You'll be drawn repeatedly to a certain key. In my own development, the key I've been drawn to most in the Western scale is D. It evolved as the pivotal key around which I composed many songs in the early years of the previous decade."

Professor Will Johnson, anthropologist and mystical seeker, reports a parallel experience. "I was in the Sierras in the open country, hiking alone for about ten days and I noticed that my voice came out (that usually didn't happen), and I sang all kinds of things. I noticed that as soon as I got home I stopped singing again. It was a rather jarring effect." At present he's recovered his vocal capacity.

The serenity that reveals itself in silence grants permission for musical expression.

Meditation

Volumes have been written on meditation. Most people are mystified by all the talk surrounding it. Yet, all that is needed is to allow yourself to meditate. We are all natural and capable meditators. It's just that the endless methods spoken and written about it tend to inhibit the flow we have with it. Once we take the time to sit in silence, we discover the inner world and the Divine connection. I have found major breakthroughs for novice meditators and long frustrated ones using these simple techniques.

There is a stage where endless chatter goes on in the mind. Let it pass without following the thoughts anywhere. They'll run on until they run out and then comes the wonder of silence upon Silence.

There are times when meditation is filled with visions and insight, and others when it's magnificent stillness once again. In that silence, you communicate with countless beings whose physical plane consciousness is momentarily suspended to blend with yours. They may be people you know and the experience is telepathic. They may be other souls you've known in past lifetimes, reconnecting for a brief interlude to say, I remember and love you. You may be uniting with guardian angels, your own spirit guides, your higher self, your Oversoul, or the Source. In all these cases, silence is the battery recharger for unconditional love.

Once in a meditative state, you are no longer aware of traffic, the telephone, and other noise. The silence of the Source calls you inside irrespective of outer discord. Although you bask in inner silence, you may respond to another human being approaching since their vibrational field sends out warning signals prior to contact being made. A Chinese Buddhist teacher once told the me that "The Mother's Meditation" is the most extensive one, for while she listens to the stillness within, she always remains poised on the physical plane, lest one of her children need her.

You might be such a deep meditator that you are unable to respond unless touched, and then you come back sharply, layer by layer. A student in a workshop described eleven states of consciousness she hurled through returning to the earth plane when someone abruptly approached her as she rested between segments of the Meditation of Water. The woman was unaccustomed to altered states. Had the man not spoken to her, she would never have realized how full and intense her meditation was.

For people who feel overcome by waves of tiredness at 4 p.m. (16:00), this is their best natural hour to meditate. Others, like myself, are early morning risers who find the silent times before the sun wakens the local population most conducive to meditation. People have reported excellent results at noontime and midnight. In that body clocks and rhythms are highly individual, notice your pattern and honor it by meditating at the hour your emotional/physical self chooses. Your downtime is the psyche's way to remind you to take time out to revitalize the spiritual/emotional body.

Breathing Awareness

Sensitive breathing is the main valve into the meditative state. When the breath is too quick, it keeps the mind from entering altered states of consciousness. For those whose thoughts run on, the exercises described here are tried and true ways to overcome resistance to meditation.

Each breathing exercise works to clear your body/mind of different conditions that inhibit meditation. Do the one(s) you feel you need, even if they are difficult to perform at first.

• Sit on your buttocks, with your legs folded in front of you, right heel against your body, left heel in front of the right calf. You may also sit with your legs folded under your body, heels against your buttocks. Or if your flexibility permits, sit in the classic yoga lotus pose.

• Exhale fully, then contract your abdomen many times. Inhalation is automatic. Repeat this process five times. This exercise gets the bowels moving. It helps the digestive process and in doing so clears the head.

• Fast, short exhalations through the nostrils continuously for up to two minutes will clear the system of mucus. Inhale completely, exhale in short, jerky sniffing sounds, as if you were having trouble blowing your nose. This exercise makes a lot of noise. In Yoga, it is called the breath of fire because it energizes the body and psyche. If your energy is too low meditation is impeded.

• Cover your right nostril with your right thumb. Breathe in through the left nostril and hold the air a moment. Cover your left nostril with your ring and pinky fingers and exhale via the right nostril. Then begin again, inhaling through the left side of your nose. This form of breathing enhances intuitive states of mind. Five minutes of slow, careful inhalation and exhalation will calm the ordinary mind and let in higher consciousness.

• This breathing practice is good for tension, anxiety, or insomnia. Lie down flat on your back, turn your palms up to relax your shoulders. Place your arms out about a foot from the body. Spread your legs wider apart than your hips. Breathe in slowly, allowing the breath to fill the abdomen first. Then bring the inhalation up to your rib cage, expanding it. Permit the air to flow upwards into your chest, shoulders, and neck. Exhale, beginning with the abdomen and ending with your shoulders and neck. Repeat this for five minutes. Breathing in this manner is so relaxing that it may put you to sleep. Once you are accustomed to relieving stress this way you'll be able to go into deep meditative states.

Quaker Healing Circle

Healings of exceptionally high quality can be done in a silence broken only by the names of the persons being cared for. Quakers

have a very powerful form of healing circle held at religious encamp-
ments and for injured or ill individuals in need of silent ministry
at other times.

The Healing Meeting is usually held at six in the morning prior
to breakfast. The chairs are placed in a circle by the conveners before
the appointed time. People seat themselves in silence. Participants
sit meditating, with all thinking suspended. From time to time
thoughts do pass through the minds of those present, but they aren't
to be dwelled upon. They are noticed and let go, although they may
relate to healing or to someone who has been named.

At least fifteen minutes of absolute quiet is maintained before
beginning to name people who require healing. The name is said
once, and silence is resumed. Further names are offered, and silence
is observed between each one. This part takes twenty to thirty
minutes with large groups and proportionally less with smaller ones.
Fifteen minutes of silence ends the hour. Only the first name need
be spoken. God knows who you are referring to, for each person's
name carries their vibration with it even if it is a very common one.

At a bedside gathering people sit around the person in silence
and if someone is inspired to speak they do so briefly. It is most usual
that the entire gathering be silent. People speak when the Spirit
moves them. Meetings for healing may also be held without the sick
person present. In that case, the group congregates either in the
Meeting House or at someone's home. The procedure is the same.
The presence of God or the Holy Spirit is felt in increasing volume,
in direct relation to the depth of silence in the room and the unifica-
tion of individual consciousness into one.

Silence: A Very Special Way To Worship

A Western form of meditation which allows for judicious speech
is silent worship as practiced by The Society of Friends. Gathering
in silence, broken only by inspiration so deep, you shake with force,
indicating that your vocal ministry is wrought by the Holy Spirit,
or the Light. When a Meeting is truly gathered, the silence is very
moving. Thoughts traveling through an attender match those of
others in the room. Speakers who rise and break the silence to deliver
a message to Meeting speak to the condition of others present. The
speech is short, pointed, from the heart, and unpremeditated.
Silence resumes. If another person feels moved to speak, they rise

and address the Meeting. Following their message, the silence continues. The silence holds all present in a common bond of unity and grace.

You can worship in the manner described whether or not you are of the same persuasion as the Friends. The method is empowering and gratifying. Sit in any comfortable position. You and your friends can preset a time limit for your meeting, or you may end when you all feel moved to. The room should be uncluttered and pleasant. If meeting out of doors, make certain that the weather isn't disturbing such as fog, excessive wind, heat, or chill. Follow the form described above, remaining respectful of one another and inviting the presence of the Creator with your silence.

Inner Quiet

There are many mysteries that inner silence reveals. To know what they are, you have to take the trouble to explore the quiet space that holds the stillness inside the core of your very being. Once you know the inner quiet, you shall seek it over and over, for that is the deepest well of renewal and reconciliation sentient beings can go to. In that place, in ourselves, we know God. We are One.

Prayer

Native Americans believe prayer must be said out loud because your voice and your breath must place your vital force into action to make something happen. Your voice contains vibrations that are yours alone. Molecules shake and realign themselves from the energy released by the sound of your voice. That does add power to praying.

If you are in a situation where you cannot pray aloud—a hospital room, a chapel occupied by other people, your place of work—pray silently. The Source knows every thought, every impulse. Your sincere prayer will be heard, even when you pray in silence. No grandiose words are needed. Your own commitment, your own fervor is the only requirement.

Following prayer, let your thoughts on the matter rest. Praying once an hour over the matter at hand is always helpful in circumstances of life and death or severe mental anguish, but let your mind remain free of the burden between times. Excessive concentration on someone or something can overload the mental, spiritual, and emotional circuitry. Once you turn a situation over to the Creator, trust God to take care of it. A prayer is never unanswered, but often the reply isn't delivered in exactly the manner we prayed for. The Universe always reveals the way which points to our highest good. Our choice is either to accept what we're given and do it gladly or feel rejected and angry because it's not precisely to our liking.

Diana Lampen in her book *Facing Death* (Quaker Home Service, 1979), writes, "We may not have what we call an answer at all; though we can always look at it like the little girl did who prayed for fine weather for her outdoor birthday party. When it rained, some said, 'God didn't answer your prayer.' She answered, 'Oh yes, he did. He said No.' "

Some of the finest healers in the world are able to affect cures with prayer alone. Their trust in the Creator is so strong that they have a direct line to the Creator's ears. When your prayer is answered exactly as you wished, remember to give a prayer of thanksgiving. If it is not, pray harder and say thank you for the lesson you have received.

Peace

The answer to creating world peace lies within ourselves. The breath that gives us life is the key to peace. When we are anxious or upset, a few deep breaths serve to calm us; to sing, we must breathe deeply for the notes to be held. A song is a prayer set to music. Placing the power of our heart's desire in song and words creates the reality we want. The militaristic elements in our society have sung in groups for centuries, celebrating past victories and the glories of war. The technique has worked perfectly to keep the world in turmoil. If we want peace, we must give up commemorating and honoring wars and battles.

The farmers, fishermen, and schoolteachers of Surray, Maine went to Russia in 1986 as the Surray Opera Company. They spent their own money to reach the citizens of Russia via sound. They'd painstakingly learned "Boris Godunov" by Moussorgsky in the Russian language. The people of one Russian city were so impressed that they accompanied the Downeasters back to their hotel, singing to them through the streets. One American man from the opera said, "When you make a sound that touches another's heart, it's magic.

Words are only one way of communicating." The singers, who are just citizens like you and me, did it as a form of outreach towards the people of Russia. "When the people (of the world) get together, they can overcome the tyranny of the governments," another declared.

The keening done by the women at Greenham Common failed to alter the circumstances of war because the sounds were only a releasing method. Valuable to clear stale emotions or unbearable pain, but Wailing does not actually ask the Creator for a specific change. The Civil Rights Movement succeeded with its prayerful anthem: *We Shall Overcome.*

> *We shall overcome,*
> *We shall overcome,*
> *We shall overcome someday,*
> *Deep in my heart,*
> *I do believe we shall overcome someday.*

Singing alone or in unison with others, songs of peace and understanding containing this aspiration for our world are simple, non-violent, sacrificial offerings. Let us sing of other ways and make a fresh beginning. Playing instruments enthusiastically to accompany ourselves, we can sing out loud and strong proclaiming joyous harmony amongst the women, children, and men who comprise the world family. All-inclusive songs of sharing, loving, and interdependence can replace the separatist, nationalistic, religiously chauvinistic melodies which ordinarily send their message out into the Universe. If we are really determined to create universal peace out of the chaos we now have, the only way that will work is to be absolutely pacific in our approach. Who shall be the peacemakers? Everyone of us. For we shall literally be singing for our lives.

We are a gentle, angry people, And we are singing, singing for our lives.
We are a gentle, angry people, And we are singing, singing for our lives.

We are a justice seeking people, And we are singing, singing for our lives.
We are a justice seeking people, And we are singing, singing for our lives.

We are a land of many colors, And we are singing, singing for our lives.
We are a land of many colors, And we are singing, singing for our lives.

We are a gay and lesbian people, And we are singing, singing for our lives.
We are a gay and lesbian people, And we are singing, singing for our lives.

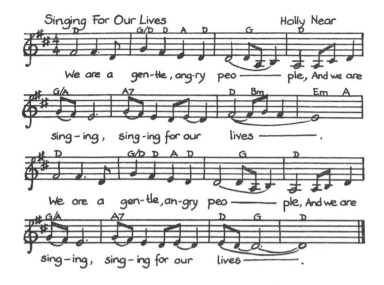

In May 1982, the peace movement sprang to life again. Throughout cities in America, people once again marched in the streets singing and chanting that the world would be one. The area of Oregon where I lived has a tremendous sense of social justice and human equality. People came in from far scattered villages, rural communities, and all the nearby cities. My daughter marched with a contingent from her high school. I joined friends from Lane County's unincorporated sections, riding our bicycles through the streets, laughing, and singing joyously with the crowd.

Entering the immense park that sits along the Willamette River, we met and cheered the Springfield marchers, and together we let out mighty roars at the South Eugene group as they entered. The excitement and exaltation was contagious. A band was playing music that proclaimed our unified minds desire to know for once in our lifetimes a world at peace.

Raptly, we hailed old friends and acquaintances we'd shared peace vigils and campaigns with in the past. But soon the speeches began, abandoning the peaceful singing for more strident verbal barrages. I turned and fled from the oral violence down to the calm of the river. Sitting there, away from the politicians, I told my friends there must be another way. "We can't out-violence the opposition, nor out rhetoric them. What is going on at the bandstand is completely from the third chakra level of power and control. If we are to create a new world order, we must move into the heart." My friends requested that I come back and listen to an elected peace politician then serving in Washington. He would be different they assured me. He was even more obnoxious and angry than the local organizers and leaders of peace groups from whom I'd swiftly run.

To the river I went once more to meditate and pray for the answer. How could we create a new movement without any violence at all? Irrespective of nationality, those in power were already such madmen; we had to use different energy to counterbalance their plutomania and hunger for world dominance. My heart weighed heavily and I left the park and the beautiful day to journey through my inner resources alone.

At the end of the week, a friend who owns a bookstore came from Portland bearing a book I'd requested she special order for me, as a reference about esoteric yoga breaths. We visited until 2 a.m. when I retired to my room with the book. First I looked up the material I'd been waiting for. And then on whim, I turned to just any page to see what it might say to me.

"Baba, how can we create peace?" The devoted student asked. "To create peace, sing, and chant unto God." (Baba Hari Dass, *Silence Speaks: From the Chalkboard of Baba Hari Dass*, SRI Rama, 1977.)

As I wrote this book in Switzerland, Holland, and England, it became apparent to me that the promise I had made to myself and the Universe when my children were young had to be fulfilled. I would take whatever risks were necessary at any personal costs willingly. I wrote to my friends:

This is not the world I planned to turn over to my children and yours. Now I know the fourth part of my Life Vision (1972) must not be ignored. Contemplation is needed to approach a truly evolutionary method of spreading peace and love worldwide. We can eradicate hunger, one of the three major flaws of the material plane. This will remove much suffering. War and disease remain; only radical alterations in our thought patterns can actually bring lasting health and peace.

Without children to raise, I can take the risks involved. Only my own life is at stake. I'm going to pray long and hard over this mission. It must be done with utmost care. There's a plan to do a worldwide meditation at 1 p.m. Greenwich time on December 31, 1986. It's being promoted widely in Europe's alternative healing community. Yet I am certain that sporadic out-pourings of this kind aren't sufficient to dismantle the war machine.

Back I came to Northern California to write, meditate, fast, and pray. On sacred Pomo ground in the closing days of the year, the prayers became a reality. The helping spirits delivered the sound for world peace. Softly sung 12 times, it will take you to the place where peace can be found. *Ahhhhh*

Sing it. It's Sound Medicine.

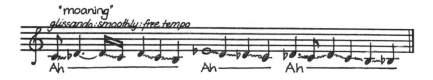

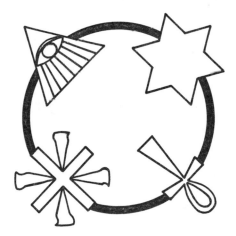

A cassette tape to accompany the songs and other material in Sound Medicine is available for $12.00 post paid, from:

Inward Journeys
P.O. Box 1112
Ashland, OR 97520

Make checks payable to: Inward Journeys.

GLOSSARY

Aphonia - Loss of voice.

Asana - Pose, position.

Creation Realm- Where human beings dwell when we are not incarnated. We go to this non-physical place during dreams and trances. Members of the angelic order also reside here.

Divine Proportions - PHI ratio of one to 1.618. If you have a window or room made in these proportions, it is more pleasing than most constructions. Our foot is a sacred number related to the earth's circumference. If you cut the pyramids vertically, at the base the hypotenuse of the triangle will be 1.618.

Glossalia - Speaking in Tongues. The person in a trance state is supposed to be communicating with spirits.

Journeying - A trance state in which you travel to other planes of existence and receive knowledge from the Source.

Healing Song - A song belonging only to you with which you heal yourself and others.

Karma - Intention, or pre-ordained situations in life. There are two types: destiny, and the pay off for our current and past behavior intentions.

Kundalini - Circular power. A spiral of energy circulating throughout the body. When it is firs awakened, it feels like flashes or waves of overwhelming heat.

Lifesong - The song the Creator gave you prior to birth: it is your power song.

Mantra- The uttering of sacred sounds.

Nada- Iinner sounds.

Overtones- A method of healing with vibrational sound.

Physical Realm - Our earthly plane of existence.

Plutomania - Materialistic greed, wealth addiction.

Prana - Life force, breath.

Signal Song - A written piece of music that heralds changes or signals events in the life of an individual or a group.

Sound Wave - Sound and light are differeing emanations of frequencies. Light waves travel at a set 186,000 feet per second. Sound waves vary by the substance (e.g. water, brick) they are traveling through. They are the same energetic form, but we perceive them through our eyes or ears as different. Other parts of our body feel sound as vibration and light as color or heat.

Sucking Doctoring - A method of healing wherein the healer sucks the poison or negative force out of a person while the healer's mouth may or may not touch the person during the healing. The toxin is always spat out of their mouth.

Svália   Sanskrit word for Toning.

Synesthesia - The blending of two or more senses; sight/sound/taste/touch/smell.

Tinnitus - Sound emanating from the ear. Diagnosed as a disease, it is actually the Nada being heard by spiritually untrained people.

Toning - A method of healing with vibrational sound.

Tumo - The art of healing the body with inner fire.

Universe - All That Is. The Godforce. Collective consciousness.

zDzogChen - The core teaching of Tibetan Mysticism.

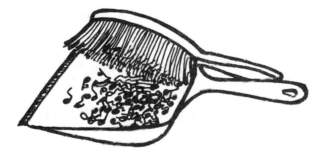

BOOK LIST

Being Peace, by Thich Nhat Hahn, published by Parallax Press.

Companions in Spirit, by Laeh Maggie Garfield and Jack Grant, published by Celestial Arts 1984.

The Cosmic Crystal Spiral, by Ra Bonewitz, published by Element Books.

A Difficult Decision: A Compassionate Book About Abortion, published by Crossing Press 1986.

Facing Death, by Diana Lampen, published by Quaker Home Service 1979.

Gemstones in the Geological Museum, by W.F.P McLintock, CB DSc. published by Her Majesty's Stationary Office (London), is not about healing but has the most complete information concerning the composition of gemstones, how they are tested, and where they are found. Written for the layman, it is an articulate and valuable reference for the stone collector. It may be purchased for £1.95 from the Geological Museum, Exhibition Road, London SW72 DE. Shipping costs are extra; inquire prior to purchase so that you can send money for the book and its delivery at the same time.

The Healing Clay, by Michael Abehsera, published by Citadel 1986.

Healing With Crystals and Gemstones by Daya Sarai Chocron carefully lists stones by their color, and outlines the way each one assists our spiritual transformation and how it heals us. Samuel Weiser, Inc. publisher.

Healing Stoned, by Julia La Russo and Joel Glick, covers all sorts of gemstones and precious metals. I've been recommending it for more than ten years. Published by Brotherhood of Life.

Healing Yourself, by Joy Gardner. The little yellow book found in more than 100,000 households as a handy reference. Crossing Press, publisher.

Healing Yourself During Pregnancy, by Joy Gardner. Filled with excellent information about maintaining a healthy body to support your healthy baby. Discusses issues your allopathic doctor doesn't know much about. Crossing Press 1987.

The Herb Book, by John Lust. Bantam 1974.

I Ching Workbook, by R. L. Wing, Doubleday & Co. 1979.

The Magic of Precious Stones is a superbly readable, extremely practical book by a highly recognized Dutchwoman, Mellie Uyldert. Published in England by Turnstone Press, it is as vital in the translation as in the original.

Maria Sabina Her Life and Her Chants, by Alvaro Estrada, Ross Erikson Inc.

Modern Herbal, Jeanne Rose, Putnam 1987.

Music, by Sufi Inayat Khan, Samuel Weiser.

The Music of Man, by Yehudi Menuhin, Simon and Shuster 1979.

The Mysticism of Sound; Music; The Power of the Word; Cosmic Language, by Hazrat Inayat Kahn, Servire BV Netherlands, publisher, 1979.

The Name Game, by Christopher T. Anderson, Simon and Shuster 1977.

Proven Herbal Remedies, by John H. Tobe, first printing 1969.

Through Music to the Self, by Peter Michael Hamel, published in England by Compton Press, and Element Books USA.

Toning: the Creative Power of the Voice, by Laurel Elizabeth Keyes, DeVorss and Company, publisher.

Trivializing America: The Triumph of Mediocrity, Norman Corwin, Lyle Stewart, 1986.

Women of Wisdom, by Tsultrim Allione, published by Routledge Paul P/C 1984.

INDEX

Prayer 3, 29, 54, 79, 149,
  150, 166-67, 171
Primal Sound 133, 135
Primary Channel 41
Problem 131, 132
Protestant 79
Psyche 21, 77, 90
Psychic Attacks 118
Purification 30, 44

Quaker Meeting 82
Quakers 164-67
Quartz 113, 115, 116, 117,
  118, 121-25

Racism 32
Radio 31, 54, 55, 87, 89
  90, 91, 99
Radioactivity 137, 138
Realm of Creation 45
Records 15, 33, 101
Recording 33, 92, 102-12
  Binaural 103, 107
  Digital 107, 108
  Tape 102, 107
Refrigerator 88
Religion 31, 32, 72
Religious Buildings 57, 66
Resonance 65
Rhythm 36, 37, 40, 131
Ritual 49, 50, 53, 149
Roan, Neill Archer 42
Ruby 113, 115, 118
Runes 136
Russia 167, 168

Saint 124
Sapphire 113, 115, 118

Sanscrit 19, 45, 56, 97
Scale 37, 38
Seawater 149, 151
Secondary Channel 41, 42
Second Languages 18-21
Secret Sound 51, 56, 82
Senses 9, 21
Shamanism 3, 5, 128-38,
  139
Shaman 5, 114, 128-38,
  139, 162
Sharp 38, 39
Signal Song 48, 54, 55
Silence 3, 11, 71, 76, 89, 90,
  93, 138, 153, 154, 160-62,
  164, 165-66
Singing 150
  Animals Responding 24,
    25, 129
  Bowls 128, 132, 135
  Driving While 24
  Harvesting 28, 29
  Medicine 14
  Memory 15
  Over food 30
  Peace 168-71
  Purification 30, 43
  Spiritual 14
  To Spirits 25
Sinus 118
Sixties 32
Smell 3, 9, 73, 91, 105
Smoking 17, 28, 29, 96, 148
Sonar 95-97
Soprano 4, 58, 59
Sound
  In Nature 93, 102, 103, 105
  Library 101-12
  Man-Made 101, 102, 104,
    105, 107, 108-12
  Pain 8